YOU CAN CURE CANCER AND LIVE THIRTY YEARS LONGER

FRED TESSLER

First edition

Copyright @2017 by Fred Tessler
Edited by Lotte and Robert Tessler
Cover Image: **Mona Lisa** by Leonardo Da Vinci
Cover Image: **Fruit Still Life** by Peter Dee
Peter Dee: http://www.peterdee.ie/
Cover Design: Robert Tessler
Layout & Typography: Robert Tessler

All rights reserved. No part of this book may be reproduced or transmitted in any way or by any means, electronic or mechanical, including photocopying, recording and information storage and retrieval systems, without the written permission of the publisher, except where permitted by law

ISBN-13: 978-1974660070

ISBN-10: 1974660079

Please visit Fred on the web at http://www.fredtessler.com
Facebook: http://www.facebook.com/fred.tessler.7

DISCLAIMER

Please note that all health information contained in this book has been sourced from existing medical knowledge with the exception of prostate problems, improved sleeping and tinnitus from which the author has suffered and after much hard work, trial and error has cured himself. Although the information and suggestions in this book are helpful it is also important that one seeks traditional medical treatment from a general practitioner.

All the information, techniques, skills and concepts contained in each chapter of this online book are of the nature of general comment only and are not in any way recommended as individual advice. The intent is to offer a variety of information in order to provide a wider range of choices both now and in the future in recognition of the fact that readers' circumstances and viewpoints will be very diverse. If any reader makes the choice to use the information contained herein, it will be his or her decision, and the author and publisher does not assume any responsibility whatsoever under any conditions or circumstances. It is recommended that the reader obtain independent advice.

CONTENTS

Disclaimer 3

INTRODUCTION 12

Getting Healthy 12

Section 1. Food and Diet 14

    Processed Food 14

    Fried Food 14

    Sugar 14

    Water 15

    Fruit and Vegetables 16

        Fruit 16

        Vegetables 17

    Dairy Products 17

    Salt 18

    Garlic 18

    Nuts, Grains and Seeds 18

    Tea and Coffee 19

    Unsaturated Fats 19

    Fish 20

    Food Combining 20

Section 2. Smoking, Drugs and Alcohol 22

    Smoking 22

Alcohol 22

Drugs 23

Section 3. Common Medical Conditions 24

Dental Health 24

Colds and Flu 24

Skin 24

Osteoporosis 25

Obesity 25

Head Aches and Migraine 25

Parkinson Disease 26

High Cholesterol 26

Candida 27

Mumps 29

Eyesight 29

Diabetes 30

Liver and Kidney Function 31

Bulimia Nervosa 31

Respiratory Disease and Asthma 31

Tuberculosis 31

Diarrhoea 32

Pneumonia 32

Food Allergies 32

- Food Allergy Tests 33
- Food Poisoning 33
- Spinal Injury 34
- Rheumatoid Arthritis 35
- Liver Damage 37
  - Symptoms of Liver damage 38
  - Maintaining a healthy liver 38

Section 3. Meditation for Healing 40
- The Technique of Meditation 41
- Visualization during Meditation 42
- Direct Medical benefits of Meditation 45
- Mental Focus 46
- How Meditation can help Drug and Alcohol addiction 47
- Additional words on Meditation 48
- Breathing Techniques 49
  - Stress and Breathing Techniques 50

Section 4. Biochemistry, Digestion and vitamins ... 53
- Digestion 53
- Biochemistry 53
- Free Radicals and Aging 54
- Toxic Overload 55
- Vitamins 57

Chromium 57

Copper 57

Calcium 57

Potassium 58

Selenium 58

Niacin 58

Vitamin A 59

Vitamin B6 59

Vitamin B12 59

Vitamin C 59

Vitamin D 60

Vitamin E 60

Vitamin K 60

Zinc 61

Riboflavin 61

Magnesium 61

Ginkgo 61

Thiamin 61

Folate 62

Lecithin 62

Iron 62

Biotin 63

- Multivitamins 63
- Herbal Compounds and Homoeopathy 63

Section 5. How to Sleep Better 65
- Biochemical solutions for Insomnia 65
- Non-Biochemical solutions for Insomnia 69
- Sleep, the Mind and Patterns of Thinking 71

Section 6. Acupressure, Healing in your Hands 75
- How to apply pressure 76
- Where to apply pressure 77

Section 7. Cancer 79
- The Causes of Cancer 79
- Why Cancer 80
- The Magic of Flaxseed Oil 81
  - How to take Flaxseed Oil 82
- Breast Cancer 82
- Colon and Bowel Cancer 83
- The anti-Cancer Diet 84
- Lifestyle changes to avoid cancer 87
- Advanced Cancer 88

Section 8. Prostate Problems 90
- Prostate Problems and Diet 92
- Importance of the Glands 94

Section 9. Sex 95

    The sexual needs of Women 95

    Advice for men 95

    Erectile Dysfunction 96

    Testosterone, Oestrogen, Serotonin, L-Dopa 98

Section 10. Suggestions for Healthy Meals 100

    Breakfast 100

        Why is this good for you? 100

    Lunch 102

    Dinner 102

Section 11. Heart Disease and High Blood Pressure 103

    What can be done 105

    How to recognize a Heart Attack 108

    The blood pressure stress Connection 109

    Blood Circulation 109

Section 12. Alzheimer's disease 112

Section 13. Depression, Stress and Panic Attacks 115

    What to do in a Panic attack 117

    Stress 120

        What can we do to reduce Depression and Stress? 120

        The danger in growing up 122

    Happiness 123

Section 14. Hearing and Tinnitus 124

    Exercise 1 126

    Exercise 2 127

    Exercise 3 127

    Exercise 4 128

    Exercise 5 128

    Exercise 6 129

    Exercise 7 129

    Improving Hearing 130

Section 15. Exercise 131

    Exercises for general well-being and state of mind 131

    Face and skin exercises 131

    Mid body exercises 131

    Exercise for Arthritis 132

    Eye Exercises 132

Towards Utopia 134

Additional information 137

    Cancer 137

    Stroke and Heart Disease 142

    High Blood Pressure 144

    Stress, Anxiety, Depression and Mental Illness 145

    Dementia and Alzheimer's 148

Sleep Disorders	149
Male Health	150
Diabetes	150
Bones and Arthritis	151
Obesity and Weight issues	151
Hearing Loss	152
Skin	152
Teeth and Gums	153
Inflammation	153
The dangers of sugar	153
Vision	153
Digestion	154
Headache and Migraine	155
Sinus problems	155
Liver and Kidney Function	155
Flu and Cold	155
General Health	156
Bibliography	160

INTRODUCTION

The purpose of this book is to transfer the latest health information with the aim to reduce pain and suffering.

At some point in our lives health becomes a major issue, especially as we get older. Maybe you have realized this already which is why you are reading this book. If you have read health books before some of this information will be familiar to you, this is because the information works! Other things will be new like my discussion prostate health, improved sleeping and tinnitus.

We are constantly bombarded by germs and viruses which are difficult to neutralize. Our air and water supply is polluted. Low levels of radiation from electrical devices attack our cells. Refined food products, especially canned foods, and the wrong fats, impact our digestive process. Tensions at work, home, and financial problems make us anxious and unhappy. On top of all this having the wrong diet over many years makes us even sicker.

In this book I would like to talk about the measures we can take introduce to improve our health make life more enjoyable.

GETTING HEALTHY

I am sure all of us would like to live to a ripe old age without getting cancer or other serious disease and be active to the very last days of our lives.

Let's now talk about how we can achieve this.

The Human body is working constantly to keep itself healthy. Unfortunately the amount of unhealthy material we are subjected to in our daily lives makes it difficult for our body to cope. We need to assist this natural process.

Our hard working cells are a wonder of nature. A single cell is so small, that it can only be seen under a powerful microscope and yet each cell performs a multitude of complex biochemical reactions. The details of these biochemical reactions are beyond the scope of this book but the steps necessary to enable these reactions to occur properly will be addressed immediately.

SECTION 1. FOOD AND DIET

Let's get right down to it and start by describing what we should and should not be eating. This section goes through various food groups and explains their benefits.

PROCESSED FOOD

Avoid all refined food such as white flour, white sugar, canned foods, margarines and all oils except oils manufactured by cold pressing, such as virgin olive oil.

Even if you eat fresh food the body still creates some toxins. However, if you regularly eat refined processed foods the amount of toxins produced will be much higher and the body's natural healing processes simply cannot cope.

FRIED FOOD

If possible grill or cook your food instead of frying it. The reason for this is that in the process of frying the temperatures can reach 150 degrees Celsius. At this temperature all minerals and vitamins will be destroyed and food loses its nutritious value. Not surprisingly, the unhealthiest food you can possibly eat is fried potato chips.

SUGAR

All sugars are unhealthy especially refined sugar which should be considered a poison. Breakfast cereals, refined foods, white rice, soft drinks, confectionary and tomato ketchup all contain excessive amounts of refined sugars.

Excessive sugar can damage the pancreas which produces insulin. Too much sugar in the diet eventually turns into unwanted fats clogging our blood vessels and arteries and elevates the level of triglyceride in the blood causing heart disease. (a nominal level of triglyceride is useful in our body as it forms a fine layer of insulation around our vital internal organs. Triglyceride is also deposited under our skin to keep our body temperature constant.)

If you have sugar cravings, which is common since sugar is addictive, try having a spoonful of honey instead, which is less harmful.

(for more information on sugar see sections on cancer, high blood pressure, Candida, diabetes and Alzheimer's disease)

WATER

The human body is 75 percent water. A human cannot survive more than seven days without water. Water is important for the prevention of disease. Drinking water is instrumental in delivering oxygen to the cells of the body and for removing carbon dioxide. Water is needed to remove friction between cartilage and connective tissues in the spinal cord. Neurons in the brain also need water to perform chemical and electrical tasks. Lack of water can result in dehydration, inflammation of joints as well head aches, kidney and muscle problems.

Try to drink at least six glasses of water per day. It is best to drink water early in the day to boost the metabolism during waking hours. Often we don't feel like drinking water but it is important that we do whether we like or not. Once you have a headache from lack of water it is too late to drink water to get rid of it. Athletes are familiar with the importance of drinking water before athletic events. Drinking soft drinks, tea and coffee is not a substitute for water.

Drinking six glasses of water each day decreases the risk of colon cancer, bladder cancer and breast cancer. Drinking water increases our metabolic rate and helps to reduce obesity. People who drink only

2 glasses of water per day run the risk of developing blood clots causing thrombosis and stroke.

Tap water has many impurities including chlorine, lead, aluminium, copper, calcium, phosphates, nitrates, sodium, fluoride, radium, arsenic and algae. In particular studies indicate that chlorine can cause heart disease, hardening of arteries, anaemia, high blood pressure, allergies and cancer of the bladder, stomach, liver and rectum. For this reason it is advisable to drink purified water only and to purchase a water purifier for home.

Water purifiers are available at most department stores. It is also advisable to eat food which is high in water content, such as salad, fruit, vegetables, fruit juices and some assorted nuts. If a water purifier is not available and there is a significant danger of bacteria in the water boil before drinking

FRUIT AND VEGETABLES

The importance of fruit and vegetables cannot be overstressed. There will be frequent references to which fruit and vegetables to take for particular medical conditions.

FRUIT

The best time to eat fruit is at breakfast. Alternatively, you have some porridge with rye or whole meal bread and some fruit juice. If possible eat fruit by itself on an empty stomach. Fruit eaten on an empty stomach is quickly digested whereas fruit eaten with other foods ferments and becomes acid. Dried fruit often has fungus on it and needs to be washed before eating. If you are hungry between meals have a banana.

Banana is a particularly important fruit. Banana reduces the incidence of stroke, stomach acidity and irritation of lining of the stomach. It contains tryptophan, an amino acid which the body uses to trigger the release of serotonin in the brain. Serotonin is a brain chemical which reduces anxiety, depression, increases brain power for complex tasks and helps better sleeping. Bananas are also rich in vitamin B6 which reduces symptoms of PMS and regulates blood glucose levels. Bananas are high in iron which is important in the production of haemoglobin in the blood and helps alleviate anaemia. Lastly, Banana is high in potassium and low in salt making it the perfect food for lowering blood pressure.

Prunes are good against cancer, heart disease, they also help to keep bones healthy. They are just as good in dried form.

Kiwi fruit is a good source of magnesium, vitamins C and E.

Apples are rich in antioxidants and help lower the risk of colon cancer, heart attack and stroke.

Strawberries have the highest level of antioxidants of any fruit and protect the body from cancer, and free radicals.

Oranges prevents cold and flu, lowers cholesterol and prevent kidney stones.

VEGETABLES

Here is a list of good vegetables:

Cabbage, Brussel sprouts, Carrots, Tomatoes, Onions, Turnips, Peas, Cucumber, Pumpkin, Radishes and Cauliflower.

Carotenes are good anti-oxidants, good against cancer, eye disorder, skin problems. Sources of carotenes are spinach, carrots, mangoes, sweet potatoes and apricots.

Vegetable deficiencies result in muscle cramps and fatigue.

DAIRY PRODUCTS

Reduce your consumption of dairy products, especially milk.

Exceptions to this are some yoghurts and cheddar cheese. The Lacto bacillus in yogurt kills all harmful bacteria.

Consumption of dairy products creates excessive acid and mucous in the body with the exception of butter and cheddar cheese. Rather than using regular milk use soy milk. Dairy products should be used in moderation as they clog the arteries.

Butter is a neutral fat and there is no harm in eating buttered bread or adding butter to steamed vegetables.

If you are sensitive or allergic to dairy products, then switch to soy milk and soy cheese.

SALT

People with high blood pressure should use as little salt as possible and then only salt with an iodine content. Ask your GP to prescribe you a salt substitute or buy sea salt from the super market.

If you are buying canned foods read the small print and avoid food with added salt. Try to use herbs and spices rather than salt, buy breakfast cereals with low salt and sodium content.

GARLIC

Garlic is nature's best anti-oxidant. It is a natural antiseptic and anti-inflammatory agent. It has anti-viral and anti-fungal properties.

Garlic destroys cancer cells, shrinks blood clots, reduces cholesterol levels and blood pressure, reduces blood clotting and the possibility of strokes, helps the immune system, aids proper digestion and reduces the possibility of Alzheimer's disease.

(see also the chapter on candida)

NUTS, GRAINS AND SEEDS

White bread is of little nutritional value. Substitute it with whole meal or whole grain bread.

Include some Sunflower kernels with your diet. Remember to wash them before eating, as most seeds have some pesticides on them.

Almonds, walnuts and all other seeds should be washed with warm water before eating. Sharply reduce the ingestion of pastas. Pasta is generally made from white flour which is an utterly useless food product and creates constipation.

Walnuts are rich in selenium, vitamin E, potassium. Walnuts can lower blood pressure, reduce inflammation, keep blood sugar levels in good balance and are rich in Omega 3 which is essential for proper brain function.

Lentils are one of the best sources of fibre, rich in calcium and folic acid.

They are very important foods for vegetarians as they high in iron.

TEA AND COFFEE

Don't drink more than one cup of tea or coffee daily.

Herbal teas are generally milder on the stomach and contain less caffeine. You can purchase herbal teas in any supermarket. The taste of some herbal teas can be improved by adding apple juice.

UNSATURATED FATS

Unsaturated fats are essential for health. Every cell in the body needs some unsaturated fat.

Saturated fats on the other hand are bad and cause over production of cholesterol. Saturated fat is contained in meat, whole-milk dairy products, including cheese, sour cream, ice cream butter and margarine. Wherever possible try to use low fat versions of these products, e.g. low fat milk and lean rather than red meat.

High cholesterol can cause cancer, stroke, heart diseases liver problems and diabetes.

The best sources of unsaturated fat are: Cold pressed Virgin Olive oil (Virgin olive oil is rich in Vitamin E and helps keep the heart healthy), Flaxseed oil, Udo's oil and Olives. These oils will increase the level of oxygen in the blood which in turn will increase our metabolic rate and help people lose weight.

FISH

Fish oil is an excellent antioxidant and source of Omega 3. Fish oil is helpful for healthy brain function. It is also useful for relieving the symptoms of arthritis and avoiding macular degeneration in the eyes. People who don't eat a lot of fish often turn to fish oil supplements in tablet form.

Wild Salmon (not from lakes) is rich in Omega 3 it helps to lower blood pressure and to reduce blood clotting.

Note however there has been some controversy over the benefit of fish oil due to high mercury levels in some fish stocks.

FOOD COMBINING

Many people try vainly to get well through a variety of diets usually not achieving the results they were hoping for.

    The reason for this is that they are eating the wrong food combination.

    For example when you eat meat followed by cake or even fruit, the meal will take six to eight hours to digest.

In fact the body will be so exhausted from digesting food that it will have little energy left for healing processes. Mixing meat and fruit together can also create internal gas which can cause a great deal of discomfort.

However, if you eat meat and vegetables together with high water content, and no sweets, it will take only four hours to digest.

Note that you should not eat baked potatoes and meat together, mashed potatoes are acceptable.

Don't eat fish and rice together, don't eat two types of proteins together such as turkey and beef, eggs and sausage. Eggs should be eaten with as little bread as possible, as mixing proteins with carbohydrate will take much longer to digest.

If you wish to eat sweets, they are best eaten three to four hours after a main meal.

It is important that fruit should be eaten separately and not mixed with other foods. Do not eat meat and fruit or sweets together, as it will take much longer to digest and it will exhaust your body. Wait for two to three hours before you have your fruit or sweets. As a rule fruit should be eaten separately. Fruit eaten on its own can be digested in one hour.

SECTION 2. SMOKING, DRUGS AND ALCOHOL

SMOKING

In the famous words of Yul Brenner; *"Don't smoke"*. Recent studies have shown that people can add as much as twenty years to their lives by simply avoiding alcohol, cigarettes and eating of fruit, vegetables and nuts.

The dangerous habit of smoking and excessive drinking is often taken up by men and women when they are young, not thinking about the future and later becomes an addiction they cannot shake.

ALCOHOL

Alcohol abuse has a long history. The link between crime, marital problems, violence, traffic accidents and alcohol goes back hundreds if not thousands of years. Our modern age is no different. Most traffic accidents which result in death or serious injuries are related to consumption of alcohol. One can often read in the media stories of horrific train or bus crashes caused by intoxicated drivers.

Alcohol is also bad for the body damaging the brain, liver and kidneys. Some people claim that moderate drinking, such as two or three glasses of alcohol are beneficial however according to the latest scientific findings this assumption is wrong.

People who drink two or three glasses of alcoholic beverages per day have a much greater chance of having a stroke than those how are satisfied with one drink with their evening meal. Alcohol is especially dangerous for young people whose brains are not yet fully developed.

Both alcohol and refined sugar are poisons. Once they get through the blood brain barrier they deplete essential glucose and water and kill large numbers of brain cells. Alcohol destroys serotonin in the brain which is essential to sleep and for control violent impulses coming from the unconscious.

Vested business interests throughout the world spend billions on advertising to promote alcoholic drinks. Whereas smoking has been widely accepted by world governments as a health hazard and advertising is restricted alcohol is still freely promoted. Alcohol addiction often begins at a young age when children feel obliged or pressured into copying their parents or peer group drinking habits.

Marriages are destroyed by alcohol abuse.

Alcohol exacerbates mental problems for people already suffering or with latent mental problems.

Alcohol causes dehydration and reduces the body's intake of vitamins which makes digestion difficult. All heavy drinkers are affected by nutritional deficiencies. It is very difficult to give up alcohol however if one decides to follow a healthy diet and cuts out refined foods and sugar it is possible.

Alcohol causes cancer of the liver, throat, and pancreas.

Alcohol is the main reason for domestic violence fire, murder and deadly car crashes. There are more heart attacks among men than women because men drink more than women.

DRUGS

Drugs, excessive drinking and smoking are decreasing the fertility rates in the western world.

Body builders are courting danger by using Anabolic Steroids, according to statistics the rate of suicide is much higher among for users.

SECTION 3. COMMON MEDICAL CONDITIONS

This section goes through various common medical conditions and explains possible solutions. Major diseases such as heart disease and cancer are dealt with in dedicated chapters later in the book.

DENTAL HEALTH

Looking after your teeth is more than just going to the dentist when you have a tooth ache. Studies have shown there is a direct link between periodontal disease and coronary artery disease, stroke, diabetes, osteoporosis, respiratory disease and gingivitis.

There is a clear link between periodontal infections and these diseases. Yet the removal of plaque which causes infection is a simple procedure which can be performed by any dentist. In an age where dental care is readily available there is no excuse for not getting a check-up every six months regardless of whether you are having obvious dental problems. Also we can perform much of this cleaning ourselves by flossing every day and using medicated tooth picks.

Bad breath comes from bacterial colonies growing in the mouth and can be a sign of gum disease. Gum disease is a precursor to losing one's teeth.

COLDS AND FLU

We all get colds and flu. If you feel a flu coming on gargle with warm salt water, drink the juice of two lemons mixed with some apple juice. Drink plenty of fluids including tea with honey.

SKIN

For people suffering from skin problems, improvement can be achieved by eating fruits rich in vitamin C. Lemon juice mixed with apple juice is also recommended. Ground nuts and sesame seeds are also beneficial.

OSTEOPOROSIS

Osteoporosis is a condition where the bones became brittle and break easily.

By eating one table spoon full of sesame seeds once a day with your meal you will reduce the possibility developing osteoporosis.

Sesame seeds are high in Calcium which is important for healthy bones. Also, include in your diet: fruit, vegetables, dairy products, sardines and lemon juice.

OBESITY

Excessive weight is directly related to heart disease, stroke and arthritis. If you are interested in controlling your weight, and you should be, then it is essential that you reduce your intake of fatty foods, especially animal fats and hydrogenated fats present in all margarines and oils. The only exception to this is unsalted butter which should be used sparingly. If you want to lose weight, start the day by drinking a glass of warm water. This will stimulate bowel movement.

For a morning snack have a slice of rye bread with a slice of cheese and a cup of herbal tea mixed with apple juice.

In the late afternoon, before the evening meal have some chopped raw carrot with sultanas. This combination will reduce your desire to eat a large meal and remove cholesterol from your intestines. Basically you should be eating a diet high in fruit and vegetables

HEAD ACHES AND MIGRAINE

Headaches are caused by food allergies, high or low blood pressure, inflammation of the arteries to the brain, muscular tension in the neck, chronic constipation, insomnia, inflammation of the jaw, toxins in the body and negative emotions such as disappointment, anger and depression

What can we do about it?

Until you feel well do not drink coffee or tea, eat plenty of fruit but not citrus fruit such as oranges, lemons, limes and grapefruits, no spicy food, no Chinese food, no avocados, no nuts. Do not eat chocolate, cheese, fried food, overly hot or very cold drinks or food. Only drink fruit juices. Eat slowly.

To avoid headaches do the following:

- No not smoke and do not drink alcohol
- Drink six glasses of water daily.
- Walk for at least an half an hour daily, go swimming whenever you can.
- Practice deep breathing exercises as oxygen shortage can also cause headaches. Practice yoga, or meditation.
- Two or three times a week take some Ginkgo tablets.
- Drinking green tea will also reduce headaches.
- To reduce migraines massage your shoulders and lower neck gently with virgin olive oil.
- Put a cold pack on your forehead.

PARKINSON DISEASE

Parkinson's disease is a degenerative condition of the central nervous system. Symptoms include shaking and slowness of movement.

A dopamine shortage can result in Parkinson disease. To reduce its impact and improve brain function take five or six omega three fish capsules every day, or a soup spoon of fish oil. Two times a week take iron tablets and Zinvit tablets.

HIGH CHOLESTEROL

Cholesterol is a white, insoluble fat made by the liver and essential for absorption of vitamin D, bile for digestion, stomach acids, oestrogen, testosterone and other hormones. However, high levels of cholesterol can cause heart disease due to fatty deposits accumulating in the arteries.

There are two types of cholesterol, HDL which is good cholesterol and LDL which is the bad cholesterol. The over production of bad cholesterol is caused by eating food rich in saturated fats present in meat and dairy foods. All foods from animal products contain some cholesterol whereas foods which are plant based do not contain cholesterol.

It is important to check your cholesterol levels at least once a year. This is usually done through a blood test. High cholesterol can not only cause heart trouble and high blood pressure but can clog up the blood vessels in the penis and make men impotent.

Cholesterol lowering foods and supplements are: fruit, vegetables, vitamins B group, E, C, E, zinc, selenium (from Brazil nuts) and Chromium.

To reduce cholesterol shred one carrot, add a handful of sultanas, a little bit of pineapple juice, and mix together. Garlic is also effective in reducing cholesterol.

CANDIDA

Candida Albicans is a tiny parasite which lives in the intestine. Normally Candida is controlled by harmless internal flora (good bacteria), however when antibiotics are taken, the good bacteria is destroyed together with the bad bacteria and Candida takes over, causing you to feel sick.

The symptoms of Candida include: Skin problems, fatigue, itching of the rectum, headaches, cramps, feeling bloated, low sex drive, mental confusion, and a white coated tongue in the morning.

This situation can be remedied by adding two spoonfuls of Inner Health Plus powder daily to your fruit juice. This powder restores good bacteria and can be purchased from any health food store. Inner Health Plus must be kept in the fridge. .

Garlic is also an excellent for reducing Candida. If eating raw garlic irritates your stomach, ask your GP to prescribe Nexium. Garlic can be also taken in tablet form. A good choice is Kyolic nystatinn tablets. Take one Kyolic tablet a day with food for ten months. Kyolic tablets are available in health food stores.

If you are worried that you may have Candida, see your doctor and ask for a food allergy test. If you are affected he may prescribe of Nizoral, Nilstat or Nystatin tablets.

If your food allergy test shows that you have Candida, then for four weeks cut out the following food products; yeast (try to buy yeast free bread), sugar, honey, mushrooms, all junk food, canned foods, dairy products. (Soya milk is ok), pickles, vinegar, cakes, sour cream, melons, grapes, dried fruit, sour kraut, tomato sauce alcohol ,mustard and buttermilk.

Eat only yeast free bread, drink at least six glasses of water a day, don't eat peanuts as they are very harmful and often coated with mound.

If you find it difficult to cut out these foods then at least have a piece of raw garlic every second day for a year or a garlic tablet every day.

Flaxseed oil, fish oil, lemon juice will sharply improve the oxygen intake of the body which will destroy bugs, yeast and Candida.

Candida and yeast are harmful in large quantities and thrive on eating junk food. Eventually the formerly not so dangerous candida parasite will mutate and it will become a cancer producing agent.

Candida and thrush can also be caused in women by wiping their bottom from back to front instead of the reverse.

MUMPS

Mumps is actually the inflammation of the salivary glands. It is most common among children. It is very contagious. If affected one should immediately see a GP.

EYESIGHT

Research has shown the necessity to keep a well-balanced diet rich in fruit and vegetables to maintain healthy eyesight and avoid problems which can lead to blindness in later stages of life.

In most parts of the world the soil is now depleted of essential minerals and vitamins present in the past in fruit and vegetables. We now need to supplement our diets to make up for the missing vitamins and minerals

Besides a diet rich in fruit and vegetables add a handful of raw almonds daily, walnuts, sunflower seeds, sesame seeds and flaxseed oil. Add to your breakfast two Macuvision tablets, one table spoonful of flaxseed oil. After diner add to a glass of apple juice the juice of one lemon. These will not only help to keep your eyes healthy but it will be beneficial to your whole body.

Add to your diet carrots, bran, spinach, nuts, seeds, corn, lettuce, tomato, peas and lemon juice. Egg yolk and broccoli contain Lutein which is needed for the eye.

To maintain good eyesight it is particularly important to eat carrots and drink carrot juice once a week.

Have a handful of walnuts daily. One handful of walnuts daily plus fish oil will prevent macular degeneration which can lead to blindness.

High blood pressure can also damage the eyes so besides the above mentioned diet reduce your alcohol intake.

Stop smoking and exercise for at least an half an hour daily. Meditate a couple times daily for twenty minutes each.

Eye degeneration which can lead to blindness becomes more frequent after the age of sixty, due to smoking, drinking, drugs and high intake of refined foods.

See an optometrist once a year to test for macular degeneration which could lead to blindness. (Also see exercises for eyesight)

DIABETES

Diabetes is a condition in which the body cannot produce enough of a hormone called insulin. Insulin is produced in the pancreas and breaks down various sugars and converts them to energy.

About one in sixty people have diabetes and it becomes more common with age. By age 70 one in twelve people are affected.

Diabetes can cause kidney failure, blindness, heart disease and stroke, bad circulation and numbness in the limbs and skin infections.

Diabetes comes in two types: type 2 diabetes, where insulin injections are not required and type 1 where daily insulin injections are required.

People who have diabetes must avoid sugar. As mentioned before a generous amount of fruit in our diet will keep us healthy. However people affected by diabetes have to be careful not to eat very sweet fruits. This also applies to people in a borderline condition.

To reduce diabetes, take the following vitamins: Vitamin C, B6, B12, D, E, magnesium, zinc, chromium, niacin and riboflavin

Foods which help reduce diabetes are: Brazil nuts (two pieces per day), lemon juice and flaxseed oil.

LIVER AND KIDNEY FUNCTION

The liver has many functions including detoxification of blood, protein synthesis, and production of bio chemicals necessary for digestion. We can't live without it.

Sweating will detoxify the body and saves the kidneys a lot of work, it is the best thing you do for your kidneys besides not drinking excessive alcohol.

BULIMIA NERVOSA

Bulimia Nervosa is a serious eating disorder which if not treated can cause death. The symptoms are starvation and the refusal to face reality in spite of the fact that one is experiencing dangerous weight loss.

A person suffering from Bulimia Nervosa is inclined to consume a large amount of food then induce vomiting.

Bulimia Nervosa requires the help of a medical doctor or a psychiatrist.

RESPIRATORY DISEASE AND ASTHMA

To reduce Asthma, breast feed babies, avoid dust, stress, tobacco, reduce fat intake and exercise as much as possible.

TUBERCULOSIS

Tuberculosis is a lung disease causing coughing, sweating and weight loss.

Tuberculosis can be deadly, and is highly contagious. It is contracted by inhaling the airborne TB bacteria from infected people.

Luckily due to the advance of medical science there are a number of antibiotics available to treat this disease. The one especially effective is Isoniazid which will kill TB gems with pronged treatment.

DIARRHOEA

Diarrhoea is often caused by harmful bacteria which produces intestinal inflammation. If it lasts for a long time then the reason could be excessive mucosa or a tumour. At times even stress can cause diarrhoea.

Consult your GP for a prescription of gastro stop.

PNEUMONIA

Pneumonia is a condition in which there is a severe infection in the lungs. Pneumonia can be the result of bacteria and viruses in the nose, sinuses, or mouth, which find their way to the lungs or germs breathed directly into the lungs or foods, liquids from the mouth into the lungs.

Pneumonia caused by bacteria tends to be the most serious. In adults, bacteria are the most common cause of pneumonia (Streptococcus).

To avoid flu and other nasty infections such as Pneumonia wash your hands and face thoroughly every time you go home to wash off the millions of invisible germs floating in the air.

To avoid Pneumonia avoid too much physical exertion while wearing wet clothing.

Two or three time a day practice deep breathing exercises for a few minutes.

FOOD ALLERGIES

According to new findings, within the next 15 years half the population of the world will be affected by some sort of food allergy.

Some people get dangerously sick if they eat peanuts, others are allergic to grains. Some people are lactose intolerant and can't digest dairy products.

There is a connection between food allergies and poor sleeping habits.

FOOD ALLERGY TESTS

I would suggest that the reader ask their doctor to do an allergy test once a year. It is a simple and fast procedure, you will find out within a week if you are allergic to milk yeast or other products.

When you receive your sensitivity test result read the report carefully.

You will find that mild allergies are marked with one star, stronger allergies ones with two stars, serious ones with three stars, and the dangerous ones with four stars.

1. Completely cut out food products marked with four stars.
2. Stay away from items marked with three stars as much as possible
3. Reduce the intake of food products marked with two stars
4. Don't worry about items with only one star

To reduce your sensitivity to certain foods cut down on refined sugars and excessive salt intake. Always look at the ingredients when buying food in the super market to see what they contain. Try to drink as much purified drinking water as possible. Just doing these things will help your body heals itself within a year.

In order to avoid food allergies to try to rotate what you eat, so that you don't repeat the same food every day. This is especially true for meat.

FOOD POISONING

Food poisoning can occur from various sources, such as harmful bacteria. Most bacteria living in your intestine are not harmful; in fact they perform a great deal of beneficial work by destroying dangerous bacteria and even manufacturing some vitamins.

Food poisoning can also come from some of the chemicals we ingest with food, as well as badly washed salads or under cooked meat, vegetables and eggs. One of the worst infections is botulism; it can cause a great deal of pain and discomfort and can result in hospitalisation.

SPINAL INJURY

Many people are confined to a wheel chair, paralysed by spinal injury, where the spinal cord has been severed or broken and no nerve messages can travel beyond the point of injury. At present medical science does not offer a cure for a broken spinal cord and severed nerves.

For spinal injury we use basically the same methods used in the hearing exercises (see hearing) however we will use our imagination to concentrate on the rear of the brain at the upper part of the brain stem. The general idea is to visualize a healing cells traveling from the brain stem downwards to the broken section of the spine, healing and adding to its length until the gap between healthy upper and lower nerve endings beyond the point of damage is bridged and a solid connection between the two is achieved.

So we start. Close your eyes and start the exercise by visualizing a massive, unstoppable number of healing and bridging cells being pushed down by a dense blue column of energy from the lower rear part of the brain stem all the way down, deeper and deeper, until we reach the point of nerve damage.

We continue doing this exercise for about ten minutes without stopping.

Now we start on the second stage by visualizing the same bluish energy column, this time saturating the broken nerve endings and causing new nerve endings to grow.

As we use out imagination and concentrate on the damaged spine, the broken spinal cord will begin to grow, getting longer and longer, until eventually the undamaged nerve endings before and after the damaged section are connected. If possible try to imagine three columns of thick laser like energy flows pushing down the healing cells.

Do these exercises for 20 minutes then stop for 30 minutes to let the brain collect more energy, then start again. Do this exercise as often as you can. Although the results might not be visible for months you will immediately notice that your brain will get stronger and give you a pleasurable sensation.

The treatment is not a physical one and some may believe that the spine cannot be cured by mental visualization alone however while medical science does not offer a cure, this method does offer the possibility of healing and pain relief.

RHEUMATOID ARTHRITIS

Steps for reducing arthritic pain:

- Practice acupressure twice daily for five minutes on each hand on all points especially on the top of your fingers. For your feet, exercise using serrated wooden rollers. (see chapter on acupressure)

- Meditate at least once daily. You will find that while you meditate arthritic pain will disappear.

- Take a warm bath and add a handful of Epsom salts to your bath water before going to bed, make sure that the water is not too hot.

- Try to swim daily, if this is not possible then walk for a half an hour.

- Arthritic pain can be reduced in intensity by changing your diet to include almonds, walnuts, salmon, sardines, all bran, eggs, fruit, vegetables, garlic, flaxseed oil, fish oil, lemon juice, banana, avocado, oranges, lentils, spinach, carrots, Brazil nuts and vitamin B12. Include in your diet the following: raw apricots or dried apricots and three table spoons of sunflower seeds daily all well washed, horseradish, yoghurt with lactobacilli, onions and lemon juice. Every day eat one piece of garlic, one vitamin C tablet, one calcium-magnesium tablet. Twice a week take 250mg of fish oil, cod liver oil and pineapple. Take one table spoon of Omega 3 flaxseed oil and herbal tea in the morning and one table spoon of fish oil after lunch.

- Take one or two tea spoons of honey dissolved in hot water. Add one tea spoonful of cinnamon. Within a couple of months you should notice some benefit. Taking a Macuvision tablets will also be very beneficial.

- Drink six glasses of water daily.

- If you work with computers sit straight don't bend over.

- Attach a heavy towel on the top of your shower frame. Holding onto this pull and stretch your body up and down one hundred times, three times a day. If you do this exercise before you go to the toilet you will find that it will help you to get rid of waste products much more easily. You can derive various benefits from this exercise. In time it will strengthen the muscles all over your body especially your back. It will reduce your arthritis and discomfort. Fat will turn into muscle. Within a few months your sexual ability will also improve. The exercise will manufacture more serotonin which will lessen tension, depression and help you sleep better.

Additional steps to reduce arthritic pain:

- Twice a day do 15 minutes of slow, mild exercise. Walking and aerobic exercises are also helpful.

- If you read make sure that your fingers are wide apart and comfortable as you hold a book or a magazine.

- When doing house cleaning, use a broom with a long handle so you don't have to bend or stretch too much.

- When writing use a comfortable position.

- If you watch TV get up every half hour or so and blink ten times.

- Always sit on a straight firm chair.

- Open your fingers firmly then slowly make a fist. Repeat 30 times twice a day.

- Stand in front of plain firm chair then, put your left foot on the chair. Lean from the waist and try to touch your toes then reverse. Do this ten times daily.

- Get a professional or family member to massage painful areas.

LIVER DAMAGE

The liver is one of the most important organs in the body. It weighs approximately 1.5 to 1.75 kilograms depending on the person. Blood is carried through the liver via the hepatic artery and portal vein.

Bile which is essential for the digestion of food is supplied by the liver. Other functions are to produce urea and substances rich in Nitrogen which assist in breaking down protein in food.

The liver stores a number of vitamins, as well copper iron, and glucose.

The liver manufactures the blood proteins: albumin, fibrinogen and globulin which are essential for the immune system to fight infections.

Bile is channelled into the small intestine, where it assists digestion.

Sex hormones are also produced by the liver, and released when needed.

Liver toxicity can occur by increased level of aluminium, which can damage the liver and reduce its ability to function properly. It can also cause sclerosis, as does a high consumption of alcohol.

SYMPTOMS OF LIVER DAMAGE

The symptoms of liver damage are: nausea, constipation, bloating, diarrhoea, bad breath, coated tongue and depression.

A blood test can detect liver damage.

MAINTAINING A HEALTHY LIVER

To reduce toxins in your liver take thistle, vitamin C, vitamin E, Niacin and Omega 3 capsules.

Sharply reduce smoking and alcohol. Go easy on anti-inflammatory and anti-fungal drugs, fats, coffee, tea, (herbal teas are OK) drink at least six glasses of water or fruit juices a day. Twice a week take multivitamin tablets, and once a week take 300 mg of magnesium and 300 mg of calcium tablets. Take one vitamin E tablet twice a week and one Zinc tablet every third day. Daily use of flaxseed oil and lemon juice mixed with some apple juice will also help to keep the liver healthy.

To keep your liver healthy, eat a lot of fruit, and vegetables, especially tomatoes, spinach, cucumbers, salads, apricots, cherries, peaches, plums, strawberries, assorted nuts, raw carrot, raw garlic, sunflower seeds.

Do not eat more than four eggs a week. Egg white is OK.

The best food to eat for a healthy liver is chicken (without the skin), duck, turkey, all types of fish including salmon and sardines, ricotta, mozzarella, and cottage cheese.

SECTION 3. MEDITATION FOR HEALING

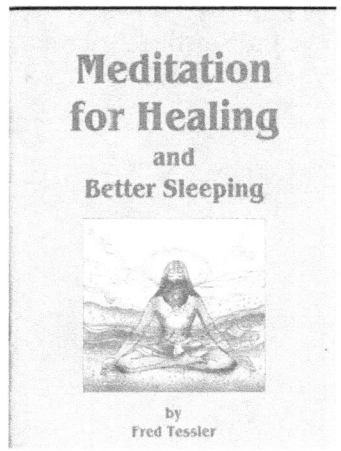

Figure 1. Meditation for Healing – by Fred Tessler

According to Indian legend the sacred knowledge of meditation was given to a select few by the God Shiva many thousands of years ago.

There have been many forms of meditation practiced over the centuries. Meditation was first practice by the followers of the Hindu religion, then by the disciples of Buddha. Later meditation found its way to Egypt and Israel. It is only in the last 50 years that the art of meditation has spread to the western world.

Meditation was introduced to the west by gurus who left India and travelled to the United Kingdom and the USA. Meditation in the western world owes its popularity to our busy life styles and the need for inner peace and balance in our lives.

To learn Indian deep meditation, pupils often had to attend classes for up to a year before they were initiated and received instruction on how to achieve perfect peace and harmony of the soul.

According to disciples, some of whom are close friends of mine, the joy of deep meditation cannot be compared to any other pleasure on Earth.

The power of the special life force that is present only in Human beings is believed by the old Indian Scriptures to be immortal and caries human experiences and knowledge across countless generations.

At the time of death, this life force, which is situated in the frontal part of the brain, leaves the body and in time enters the brain of a newborn child to live again in another person.

In the advanced state of meditation this life force radiates an incomparable quality of love that envelopes the practitioner.

In the higher levels of meditation, the life force reveals itself in the form of an intense circle of white light.

I do not wish to reveal the more advanced state of meditation. For this you must enrol in a class with a qualified practitioner. The main object of this chapter is to introduce a particular form of simple meditation that can be used to heal the mind and body.

THE TECHNIQUE OF MEDITATION

In order to achieve a perfect state of meditation all thoughts must cease.

Most people have difficulty purging all thoughts from their mind but if we use certain simple methods this can be achieved to a reasonable degree.

First, find a semi dark quiet room and a hard straight backed chair without armrests. Sit on the chair and raise both arms in front of you and shake them for the ten seconds.

Next, sit up straight with your arms on your lap and take a deep breath through the nose, hold it for ten seconds then exhale slowly also through the nose.

Repeat this procedure five to ten times.

You will probably start to yawn while doing the breathing exercises. This is normal. These exercises will help quiet the mind. We are now ready to start meditating.

VISUALIZATION DURING MEDITATION

They say that if you cannot visualize the future you cannot make it a reality. So it is with health. In meditation we visualize a solution to whatever that troubles us and let the body do the rest. Visualization opens a pathway for our body to heal itself.

For five minutes think quietly about a problem that you wish to overcome.

For example, say we have a stomach ulcer. Use your imagination to visualize billions of tiny healing cells surrounding and attacking the ulcer and replacing the damaged tissue with healthy cells. After five minutes of visualizing the eradication of the problem stop thinking about it altogether.

Now this is very difficult. However, if you continue to sit with your eyes closed and focus on your breathing most thoughts will cease.

Next become aware of your muscles becoming soft as a result of your relaxation. We chose a word or phrase, for example *"I will heal"* or *"relax"* or a simple sound like *"ahhh"* letting the last sound silently fade away as we exhale. Keep on repeating the same softly in your mind. You will find that after twenty minutes there will be fewer and fewer thoughts entering your mind.

I find it best to think the words *"ahhh"* as you breathe in and *"haaa"* as you breathe out silently in your mind.

If you find that you really can't get rid of nagging thoughts which prevent you from achieving stillness of the mind, then try singing very slowly to yourself or play classical music, operas or your favourite songs under your breath and add the words of the song with it.

Keep on doing this for forty minutes. Gradually a wonderful feeling of deep relaxation will take over your mind and body. At this stage you can stop singing to yourself and let yourself go.

In this new stillness body will heal itself faster than it would in normal sleep. The only time when the brain is really resting is during meditation.

Meditation and deep breathing will reduce your blood pressure and arthritis. It will reduce inflammation. It will improve the blood circulation and will increase the production of Serotonin, which will help you sleep better.

This method can be used for any problem. All you have to do is to change the application. The main thing is to be persistent as starting anything new is always difficult. If you keep on trying, the benefits will come. As they say *"it won't happen overnight, but it will happen"*. You may not feel the effects in a few days or even weeks, but in a month or so you will definitely feel a difference in your well-being.

Meditation can be a wonderful asset to people who are confined to a wheel chair or people with chronic migraine. At first headaches will cease while you meditate then in a year migraines will be gone. This will happen as long as you combine meditation with the diet described in this book.

Some people consider meditation a nuisance, however if you keep meditating and follow the right diet you will get better each month instead getting worse. I know some people for whom improvement of mind and body worked only after a few weeks. So if you put your heart and mind to it, then even the most chronic cases can be improved.

For example if you have been suffering from a medical or mental problem for thirty years, it can take one and a half to three years to improve your condition dramatically. I know this sounds like a long time. But the big difference is that instead of getting worse every day, you will gradually get better. For the first time in your life there is hope that you will be able to help yourself where modern medicine can't.

Try to meditate twice a day twenty minutes each time preferably before eating. If two sittings are not possible, then only meditate once a day one hour before going to bed for at least for 45 minutes.

I would like to emphasize that meditation only works if you follow some basic rules. Two hours before meditation:

- Do not drink coffee or tea.
- Do not smoke or drink alcohol.
- Do not eat red meat. Chicken, duck and turkey are OK.

The more serious the problem is the more time should to be spent in meditation.

For example in the case of so called incurable cancer a minimum of four hours of meditation is needed. However, meditation alone is not enough, good diet is also essential. Again I emphasize that besides meditation you should also consult your GP.

If you get tired sitting alone in a dark room, then find a chair in your lounge room, where the other members of your family are present. Close your eyes and think about your problem quietly for ten minutes while repeating in your mind what it is you want to achieve, then stop thinking and focus your attention on your breathing as explained previously. Do this for thirty minutes.

Of course, that will not be as effective as proper meditation but it will still be helpful.

If you are worn out and tired from a sleepless night, find a quiet place at your workplace, and meditate for 15 minutes at lunchtime. A nearby park is often a good choice.

You will find that 15 minutes of meditation will revitalize you and give you energy for the next five hours to carry on with your work.

You will notice while meditating at work or at home that you will often fall asleep for a short time. This is normal.

The few minutes of sleep brought on by meditation is worth an hour of normal sleep. So when you wake up, just continue to meditate with refreshed energy.

DIRECT MEDICAL BENEFITS OF MEDITATION

- Meditation will reduce hypertension.
- Chronic insomnia is a most unpleasant problem, which can be overcome to some degree by meditation. Results can take up to two years or be fully realized although some improvement will appear after a only few weeks. In order to sleep soundly one has to learn to relax and stop thinking about problems for which there are currently no answers.
- Pain relief

As you continue meditation, relaxation will become second nature and after a couple of years the calmness you feel will not only be present during meditation, but also during all your normal daily activity.

Many readers found it hard to believe, that a simple act like focusing on their breathing can be difficult but in fact it's not so easy. For many people it can be rather difficult to be without thoughts passing through their minds, but the art can be mastered with persistence. The main thing is not to lose patience. Don't get upset for failing at times, just shrug your shoulders, and wait for the next opportunity. It will come. Don't get discouraged if annoying thoughts persist in your mind, the healing process will still go on nevertheless.

At times you may find meditation difficult, and at other times it is easy. Keep trying, persist, think of the end result, and don't be beaten by negative thoughts.

After a long period of meditation you may find that purple or blue clouds will appear in front of your eyes. These clouds will increase in size as they come closer to you, then they will engulf you and disappear, only to reappear again later. This beautiful experience comes from the depths of your mind. Some readers might think "*who the wants to meditate for a whole year*." But don't forget that without meditation you may suffer for the rest of your life from insomnia and various other illnesses.

After a year or so, you will find that meditation will become an essential part of your life.

Here are some additional thoughts on meditation:

- Don't cross your legs while meditating, just rest your hands on your thighs.
- Don't reply to any thoughts that enter your mind.
- Do not meditate lying on a bed. It just does not work.
- If your place of residence is noisy, you can help yourself by purchasing industrial strength earmuffs or noise cancelling headphones. These will eliminate 90 % of all external noise.

MENTAL FOCUS

Most of us have a long list of problems we would like to overcome. In meditation, try to think of no more than one problem at a time.

There are a lot of people in this world who suffer from psychological obstacles to healing. A great many of these people have an in built defence mechanism that expresses itself in stubbornness, often working against their best interest. This stubbornness will come to the surface in meditation and will try to disrupt the meditative process. Let's ignore this force and put up with it while it is there. In time this force will exhaust itself.

This is why meditation not only will heal the body, but the mind as well.

Finally, I would like to point out that meditation has helped me a lot and I now could not live without its supporting comfort.

I would also like to emphasize, that meditation does not replace conventional medicine and should be used in addition to it and not as a substitute.

HOW MEDITATION CAN HELP DRUG AND ALCOHOL ADDICTION

Taking of hard drugs such as heroin etc. causes an enormous amount of pain and anguish in individuals, their families and society as a whole.

Crime is a by-product of drug addiction as addicted users will do anything to support their expensive habit.

Some claim that most drug takers are people who lack solid family background, where genuine affection friendship and security is lacking, while others state that drug takers are individuals who simply can't face the harshness of reality and find escape in the pleasure of drugs.

Some sections of the population find escape in alcohol while a smaller percentage find it in drugs. Both products are very harmful and destructive; the only difference is that drugs kill much faster.

In both cases the common denominator is escape from the harshness of life. People turn to alcohol or drugs to escape their inner fears, conflict, sadness, and worry, or sometimes just plain boredom. The individual tries to push these negative feelings aside and exchange them for euphoria of intoxication. But alas, everything has a price. Before too long the body and mind start to deteriorate from abuse.

I know a number of former hard drug users who started looking for an alternative solution when they realized their predicament. They found it when they learned to meditate. Over the course of time their feelings of inner turmoil gave way to peace, harmony, inner spiritual strength and pride in themselves. Through the years that followed they were transformed into different people and found new inner strength. They ultimately found that meditation often gave them a pleasurable feeling superior to drugs. It uplifted their spirit and they went on to lead full interesting and creative lives.

This is not to say that meditation is an escape from reality. It is a natural process of achieving calm and promoting healing necessary if we are to stay healthy.

ADDITIONAL WORDS ON MEDITATION

As mentioned previously real meditation starts when thinking and thoughts stop. When the mind is full of schemes and thoughts brain energy scatters, but when focusing on a point, wholeness is achieved and fragmentation is eliminated.

When deep meditation is achieved, our mind and brain is changing and improving, and progressing toward a better intellect and health, harmony within ourselves and creativity will follow.

After some years of meditation, our mind will open up and give us additional knowledge. The stronger the individual's enthusiasm coherence and clarity in visualizing things, the deeper the change will be in the sub-consciousness and in the mind generally. According to the great thinkers the universe and its contents is made up of the thoughts of the creator rather than real solid matter. This is a deep philosophical viewpoint lost on many but rings true if you consider that all experience come from the self.

It is believed by great thinkers that God created and keeps on creating matter by merely thinking about it. If you have ever read any articles on quantum physics you will recognize this concept. At the microscopic level matter is constantly appearing and disappearing with no explanation.

Human beings don't have the ability to create matter, but they do have the spark of a divine gift with which they can marshal their body forces, with the help of their imagination, and with a combination of their will, enthusiasm, and persistence. Prayer combined with meditation will bring a change for the better.

If one keeps meditating then eventually lethargy, depression headaches will be less and less as time goes by.

BREATHING TECHNIQUES

In the first part of the book we emphasized the importance of meditation. We went on to talk about insomnia and the possibility of curing it with the help of meditation and the right diet. We then strengthened our chances of keeping healthy by practicing the pressure treatment once or twice daily.

Now we will enlarge our knowledge by introducing breathing techniques.

This knowledge is also thousands of years old and a well-known part of Yoga exercises. These breathing exercises enlarge the lungs by supplying more oxygen to the brain and internal organs. In the long run this will not only calm your mind, but also restore youth and vitality.

The breathing exercises should be practiced where the air around you is reasonably clean. The duration should be at least ten minutes a day.

Go for walks whenever it is possible and while you walk unhurriedly practicing the various breathing exercises.

The exercises are listed below:

- Inhale slowly through your mouth, then blow the air out very fast, Repeat ten times.

- Close your left nostril with your finger while you take a deep breath through your right nostril. Hold your breath for four seconds, and then exhale through your right nostril. Now reverse the process breathing in through the left nostril, holding your breath for four seconds and breathing out.

- Take a deep breath with your mouth wide open. Hold your breath while you count to five, then, exhale slowly. After you exhaled, take another breath and hold your breath for the count of five again, then exhale. Repeat ten times.

- Close your mouth, and take a deep breath through your nose. Hold your breath till the count of five, then, exhale slowly. Repeat this ten times or more.

The ideal place to do these exercises is while walking in nature and taking in fresh air. However if this is not possible, then practice them at home. Alternatively, take a few minutes off at work and practice breathing and pressure exercises there.

I just want to add a few words. I would like to urge you to give all the described techniques a go, as it will not cost you anything except a little time. And in the long run it will help considerably to keep you healthy and make you feel better.

STRESS AND BREATHING TECHNIQUES

The breathing exercises are a perfect treatment for stress. If you are stressed, then do the breathing exercise for at least an hour or longer will work like a charm.

When we discussed meditation for healing I pointed out that before we meditate for healing purposes, we use our mind and imagination to think about our problem for about five minutes before we proceed with meditation.

We can also use other healing methods while we travel in a bus or train, or when we just sit at home in a comfortable chair and start our deep breathing exercises.

We focus our attention on the part of our body which we want to heal or improve. In breathing, exhale with eyes your closed and send your breath to the part of our body which is sick, or which you want to improve. With our exhaling breath we reinforce our tissues. We send our breath in a plain form or color, with blue, green or purple, as we wish. I know this sounds vague but visualization is a very powerful part of healing. In healing as in other things if the result cannot be visualized or imagined then there is no road to travel down the get there.

We can also use the same method for relaxation in bed when we want to go to sleep. We just breathe comfortably and send our breath on exhaling first to our toes, then to our legs, working our way up to our calves, thighs, abdomen, chest, neck and face, relaxing each set of muscles in turn with each breath. By using this technique many of us will find that drowsiness will come over us and we will fall asleep easily.

There is another breathing technique while in bed in which rather than visualizing breath traveling to parts of the body we visualize nature and a visual representation of our breath.

First let us imagine that we are sitting on a rocky hill overlooking a wide river flowing toward the lowlands. Watch the river for a short while then send your exhaling breath toward the river. As you do this the river first becomes red in color. Keep watching the red color for a minute or two, then let the color change, to light yellow, then to orange, to be followed by green, then purple, and finally to lilac, each color lasting a minute or two. This exercise can also help you to go to sleep.

SECTION 4. BIOCHEMISTRY, DIGESTION AND VITAMINS

DIGESTION

Digestion begins in the mouth where food is shredded and mixed with saliva. It is very important to eat slowly and give our saliva a chance to pre-digest food.

In the next stage food makes its way through the oesophagus, a tube well supplied with muscles which squeezes the food down to the stomach where special glands release gastric juices which digest food.

Water and alcohol is absorbed quickly from the stomach, while the remaining food must be properly digested.

After digestion food is transferred into the small intestine where various enzymes and bile break down the fats and proteins as well as the starches. Once digested and separated food will move down the length of the small intestine where digestion will be completed.

Next the various nutrients will enter the blood stream.

Food that can't be digested such as the skin of fruit and excessive roughage and mucus becomes faeces, which makes its way slowly to the end of the colon from where it will be expelled.

The exercises mentioned before will considerably speed up the rejection of faces, for if it stays many days inside the colon, will give rise to various diseases including cancer of the colon.

BIOCHEMISTRY

The body consists of approximately 30 Trillion cells; each cell is surrounded by a membrane. Individual cells accept only as many nutrients as they need, the rest such as fats keep on circulating in the blood steam until they are needed. Fats are also stored in the liver which coverts them into Bile which in turn is needed for digestion. Some cholesterol is important for the manufacturing of Vitamin D, Bile, stomach acids, Oestrogen, and Testosterone. Enzymes are special proteins manufactured by the body; one of their tasks is to aid digestion. Food is digested in the small intestine where as a rule the body only lets substances enter the blood stream which are useful.

The natural biochemical process of digestion breaks down then the body is overloaded with the wrong type of food or too much food.

FREE RADICALS AND AGING

Free radicals are unpaired electrons which attack the DNA and alter the genetic material of cells. Damaged DNA cannot replicate itself correctly and errors in cellular replication multiply or cells simply die.

The long term result of exposure to free radicals is aging, arthritis, atherosclerosis, Alzheimer's disease, cataracts, macular degeneration, diabetes and cancer.

The telomeres at the ends of DNA strands are particularly susceptible to damage. In theory if DNA could always replicate itself perfectly we would not age, new cells would be exactly the same as old ones. Free radicals have their sources in oxidants and radiation.

Antioxidants are the obvious choice for combating excessive oxidants in the body. Over exposure to the sun is a source of radiation and can cause skin cell damage and skin cancer. To further reduce exposure to free radicals reducing alcohol intake, stop smoking and stick to a healthy diet as described in this book.

To destroy free radicals add to your diet a fruit, vegetables, assorted nuts, vitamins A, B, E, 2 grams of vitamin C powder, two pieces Brazil nuts daily, zinc and magnesium. After dinner add to a glass of apple juice the juice of a whole lemon.

TOXIC OVERLOAD

The body is a fantastic self-repairing machine constantly trying to protect itself from the damaging effects of air and water pollution, alcohol, tobacco, impurities in food, some medicines, a long list of parasites, microbes and viruses.

A huge amount of energy goes into this detoxification process. Anything we can do to help our body, and take some of the burden off, will liberate surplus energy and increase our wellbeing and vitality.

As the years roll by, the body accumulates enormous quantities of toxins from the large number of dangerous chemicals present in our food and water supply, as well as from air pollution. These toxins accumulate in the mucous linings of the intestines, the stomach, in the throat and the nasal passages. They place a huge burden on the body's natural healing process and make us sick.

Although the level of infectious diseases has sharply declined in the modern world the incidence of diabetes, heart attacks and strokes has increased due to the lack of exercise and the consumption of refined foods such as white sugar, white flour, rice and margarine.

Although our body is working day and night to reduce the amount of accumulated toxins it is only partially successful.

Various poisons are stored in the liver, kidneys, in the mucous linings of the intestines, stomach, lungs and throat. The above mentioned exercises and diet will help eliminate these toxins and put us on the road to health.

We live in a toxic world full of viruses and bacteria. Apart from natural bacteria there are at least 50,000 man-made chemicals present in drugs, herbicides, food additives, farming fertilizers and industrial chemicals which we are exposed to on a daily basis. Children are particularly susceptible to infection since they are still developing immunity. The use of artificial coloring and additives in our food is unnatural and puts a further strain on the body.

There are however simple ways to protect ourselves from bacteria such as washing your hands after you go to the toilet or after you have been out in a shopping center or visiting friends. One can even get nasty diseases even from fruit and veggies, unless they are washed thoroughly. To protect ourselves from the risk of food poisoning should be cooked at least at 80 degrees Celsius (160 Fahrenheit) to kill off any dangerous bacteria.

The following anti-oxidants will eliminate accumulated poisons such as lead and mercury now often found in fish:

- Vitamin C powder
- Vitamin E
- Selenium and magnesium. e.g. Blackmore's Bio Magnesium tablets.

Some people suffering from allergies can be seriously affected by after shave lotion. So as far it is possible stay away from it.

Dirty filters in air-conditioning units are another source of pollution and bacteria. Bad air can result in the development of chronic respiratory diseases such as asthma, bronchitis, hypersensitivity pneumonitis, headaches, dry eyes, nasal congestion, nausea, fatigue and legionnaire's disease.

Overuse of antibiotics can weaken the immune system. The same damage can occur by having too many different medications over a long period.

VITAMINS

In order to rid ourselves of toxins we need to include vitamins and minerals in our diet.

Also, since most of our food products often lack essential minerals and vitamins it is necessary to get extra vitamin supplements in a pill form.

Note that it is important not to take too high doses of vitamins as excessive amounts can make you sick. So please don't overdo it.

Note: a quick way to make up for mineral deficiency is by using biochemical salts. These will restore badly needed minerals in the body. The normal dosage is one to three tablets twice a day 15 minutes before or after eating. Put the tablet on your tongue and let it dissolve, with no water added.

CHROMIUM

Chromium is useful against diabetes, heart disease.

Sources: beef, liver, whole wheat, eggs, bran, ham, raw brown sugar, cheddar cheese, spinach, corn, potato and milk powder.

COPPER

Copper is needed for good health and reduces diabetic conditions.

Sources: walnuts, sesame seeds, sardines, chick peas and avocado.

CALCIUM

Calcium is important for healthy teeth and bones and preventing osteoporosis. Calcium is also important for muscle development, reducing blood pressure and preventing cancer. Taking a calcium magnesium combination supplement is a good idea

> **Sources:** All the calcium you need can be found in milk, cheese, walnuts, soya beans, salmon, sardines, spinach, yoghurt, Brazil nuts and walnuts. (Sesame seeds are particularly high in calcium).

POTASSIUM

Potassium will reduce high blood pressure.

> **Sources**: Potato, avocado, bananas, prunes (well washed) avocado, orange juice, milk, strawberries, mango, cream of tartar, apricots, cooked beets, brussel sprouts, oranges, pears, nectarines, dates and figs.

SELENIUM

Selenium is needed to prevent cancer and aid liver function. It helps the heart, protects the eyes against cataracts, destroys blood clots and relieves arthritis. Selenium neutralizes heavy metals such as lead, cadmium and mercury which we absorb from sea foods, water and other various food products.

> **Sources**: Brazil nuts, eggs, tuna, pink salmon, turkey and bran.

NIACIN

Niacin fights depression, Alzheimer's, anxiety and confusion. A Niacin deficiency can cause diabetes, depression, dermatitis and loss of appetite.

> **Sources**: Milk, egg yolk, fish, bran, avocado, bananas,

dark grapes, apples, beef, lamb, nuts, whole grains, liver, dates, figs and prunes. Niacin can be taken in tablet form: dose 15mg.

VITAMIN A

Vitamin A is needed for healthy skin, eyes and to avoid thyroid problems.

> **Sources**: Sardines, bran, cod liver oil, liver, butter, dairy products, boiled eggs, mangos, raw carrots, apricots.

VITAMIN B6

Vitamin B6 is good against depression prostate problems and skin disorders.

> **Sources**: Banana, bran, avocado, dairy products, nuts, fish, eggs. B6 can be taken in tablet form. The maximum dose of B6 is 60mg daily. (not to be taken by people suffering from Parkinson's disease.)

VITAMIN B12

> **Sources**: liver, kidneys, whole grain, nuts, eggs, milk.

VITAMIN C

Vitamin C helps to prevent cancer, cataracts in the eye, high blood pressure, infections and diabetes. Vitamin C kills cancer cells and microbes. It will prevent heart attacks and stroke. it is vital for the immune system and is a very good anti-oxidant. It will help against cancer, heart disease and is necessary to covert tryptophan to serotonin which is needed to sleep better. Vitamin C reduces high blood pressure, prostate problems, stomach cancer, lung cancer and is needed for the eye. It will help the reproductive system. Serious lack of vitamin C will cause scurvy. To fight cancer it is essential to have Vitamin C, selenium and zinc

    Sources: The richest sources are lemon juice, red peppers, oranges, walnuts, tomatoes, lemons, strawberries, mangos, Brussel sprouts, broccoli, avocado, kiwi fruit and in tablet form, maximum dose 100mg.

VITAMIN D

Vitamin D is important for the skin and is produced by the body in response to exposure to the sun. Over exposure to the sun is not good however and can cause skin cancer.

    Sources: salami, sardines, tomato, corn, cod liver oil, pink salmon, eggs, avocado, dairy foods, vegetables.

VITAMIN E

Vitamin E is needed to create bile essential for digestion. Vitamin E will prevent heart disease, cancer cataracts, diabetes, Alzheimer's, fatigue, headaches, strokes and memory loss. It is also a very good antioxidant, good for the eyes and against Parkinson disease.

    Sources: hazelnut, avocado, spinach, tomatoes, canola oil, broccoli, grapes, hazelnuts and eggs.

VITAMIN K

Vitamin K is needed for kidney function and blood clotting.

    Sources: eggs, soya beans, broccoli, spinach, avocado, lettuce, carrots and cucumber.

ZINC

Zinc is especially important for children and pregnant women. Elderly people often develop zinc deficiency which can bring on liver disorder, diabetes.

Sources: One can buy zinc tablets at chemist shop.

RIBOFLAVIN

Riboflavin Useful against diabetes and cataract.

Sources: Fish oil eggs liver, kidney, milk, cheese, tomato, pink salmon almonds and malted milk powder.

MAGNESIUM

Magnesium is an effective supplement against Arthritis, liver disorder, Parkinson's, cancer, and an excellent anti-oxidant. A Calcium and Magnesium combination will enhance your health and help you to sleep better.

Sources: Beans, halibut, nuts, soy milk, whole wheat bread, tofu, cooked spinach, pumpkin seeds, oysters, baked potatoes with the skin, prunes, tomato and yoghurt, magnesium is also available in tablet form from any chemist e.g. Blackmore's bio magnesium.

GINKGO

Ginkgo helps brain function, reduces Alzheimer and depression.

THIAMIN

Thiamin is needed to keep your heart, nerves and brain cells healthy.

Sources: Pork, liver, lamb, seeds, peas, legumes.

FOLATE

Folate is good against Alzheimer's, as well as against depression, gut damage, cancer and hepatitis.

Sources: vegetables, lentils, oranges, avocados and tablet form: maximum in 400mcg daily.

LECITHIN

Lecithin is derived from Soya beans. 85 grams daily of Lecithin supplements can lower cholesterol levels. Lecithin keeps cholesterol soluble in bile and preventing the formation of gallstones. Lecithin converts body fats to energy more quickly and helps people lose weight.
Lecithin improves memory and is frequently taken by elderly people and those suffering from Alzheimer's disease, dementia and Parkinson's disease. Lecithin comes in granular form and can be taken up to three tablespoons daily.

Sources: cold pressed vegetable oils, egg yolk, nuts and seeds.

IRON

Iron is an important mineral for combating Parkinson's disease, Alzheimer's and to maintain a health liver and prostate. It is particularly important for women to maintain their iron levels. Iron is also helpful for reducing general anxiety.

Sources: Eggs, banana, melon, lamb, chicken, Spinach, lentils, seeds, beans, tomato, fruit, dried fruit, potatoes, liver, salmon, tuna, poultry and oysters.

For Vegetarians: Lentils, oats, cooked spinach, and

chick peas cooked, almonds, raisins, apricots and cooked beans.

BIOTIN

Biotin will help the immune system produce white blood cells.

Sources: corn, milk, peas, liver, hazelnuts, eggs, chocolate.

Almonds Brazil nuts (3 pieces daily) lemon juice, magnesium will repair internal cell damage.

MULTIVITAMINS

Obviously there are a lot of vitamins out there. For this reason many people take multivitamins to reduce the number of pills they have to take. Some good combinations are:

- Magnesium and calcium
- B complex
- Fish Oil and Omega 3
- Vitamin C, Selenium, Zinc and Vitamin E for preventing heart disease

HERBAL COMPOUNDS AND HOMOEOPATHY

Although often homoeopathic medication work when everything else fails, some people may react to them in a negative way, in which case discontinue the usage.

Arnica: assists skin and bone healing process. After a bad fall take Arnica ointment twice daily.

Calcarea Fluorata: is used to heal ulcers, decaying teeth, goitre as well as blurred vision, damaged muscles, cataracts. Calcarea Fluorata sulfur is a great cell healer, effective against skin problems and slow healing wounds.

Calcerea Phos: will speed up bone healing, excellent against leg cramps ,back pain and stomach disorders.

Kali Mur: is used to treat Asthma, it helps to form new brain cells, it is good against rheumatism and strokes. It is effective against hay fever, stomach problems, constipation. Natrum Mur to heal headaches.

Kali Phos: is essential for the proper working of the brain, blood, nerves and muscles. Deficiency of this mineral will brings nervous disorders, sleeplessness, indigestion, and depression.

Ferum Phos: is essential for the body to form red blood cells. It is also helpful against inflammation, rheumatism, kidney and bladder problems and it helps the general healing of the body.

Lycopedium: is useful in case of lost sexual desire, impotence, insomnia, loss of hair and depression.

Echinacea Purpurea: is excellent to fight infection, it boosts the immune system of the body .It stimulates the production of infection fighting white blood cells. It also reduces the size of internal tumour's. It is also useful against flu, sinusitis, ear infection, urinary infection, skin problems and allergies.

SECTION 5. HOW TO SLEEP BETTER

Sleep is a most precious commodity especially appreciated by those who don't get enough of it. Chronic lack of sleep is a terrible sensation where the unfortunate victim cannot sleep at night no matter how tired they are. For a person suffering from insomnia a deep peaceful sleep is the most valuable thing in the world.

According to sleep researches most people who complain about not being able to sleep, do in fact sleep at least five or six hours every night. However instead of experiencing the pleasant sensation of tiredness and sleepiness on retiring, insomniacs stare up the ceiling of their bedroom in darkness unable to get a deep restful sleep. When sleep finally does come, it comes without them noticing it. They close their eyes and fall asleep in a fraction of a second however their sleep is light and usually dreamless only lasts for one or two hours at time. They are often not aware that they have slept at all.

The next morning they get up feeling tired and miserable. They muddle through their day dogged by exhaustion and nagging discomfort. When the time comes to go to bed again they are afraid to face another sleepless night. The ones who do manage to dream do a little bit better as they can prove to themselves that they did indeed sleep, however in spite of this they still suffer from exhaustion while at work.

Many try sleeping pills, but alas, in the long run this is unhealthy, doesn't work well and masks the real problem.

BIOCHEMICAL SOLUTIONS FOR INSOMNIA

The solution to the sleeping disorders is to restore the proper biochemical balance to the body. There may be a particular type of food or drink which upsets their sleep patterns. If the food can be identified and cut out then good sleep patterns will return. For example some people can't sleep well if they eat Chinese food. A food allergy test can identify which foods you should steer clear of.

To promote normal sleep include milk and cheese in your diet. Milk and cheese promote the production of serotonin, a brain hormone which supports sleeping. If you are on a diet, you can still drink low fat milk or eat low fat cheese. You can easily compensate for the extra fat present in milk and cheese by eating shredded carrot mixed with a few sultanas and lemon juice every day. Also add some oat bran to your breakfast food. These promote the production of bile in the body. Bile consumes cholesterol thereby cleaning the blood vessels of unwanted cholesterol.

Don't drink coffee after 4pm as caffeine will keep you awake. Drink a half of a glass of warm milk with a tea spoonful of honey one hour before bedtime.

Banana and Kiwi fruit will also help you to sleep better. If you are allergic to milk then drink a half a glass of Soya milk with two valerian tablets, one tablet of magnesium calcium combination and one B12 Vitamin tablet half an hour before bedtime. If you wake up in the early hours of the morning, take another valerian and magnesium tablet with half cup of apple juice.

As a last resort ask your GP to give you a prescription for Temaze tablets but don't take more than one of them.

Another product useful for sleep disorders is Melatonin. Melatonin is a natural product manufactured by the brain itself. You can buy Melatonin in any health food shop. One or two soup spoons of Lecithin four hours before bedtime are also helpful.

Ask your GP about vitamin B12 injections. If you have difficulty swallowing B12 tablets then crush then with a spoon and add some apple juice. B12 assists sleeping and also helps to build Myelin tissue covers to protect the nerve fibres.

Avoid eating fish or prawns especially at night, as fishing grounds are often polluted with heavy metals and can affect sleep patterns. Note that heavy metal pollution or toxins such as lead cadmium, mercury, can be neutralized with Vitamin C, E and Zinc.

Twice a week after food take bio zinc tablets.

To sleep better and burn cholesterol faster eat the following food products; eggs, liver, brown rice, almonds, avocado, lentils, roast poultry without the skin, milk and wheat germ.

It is important to have your evening meal three hours before going to sleep and don't eat big evening meals. Make lunch the main meal of the day.

One hour before going to bed have some milk and honey or the foods mentioned above with milk and honey.

Sleep disturbances can also be caused by eating meals cooked in pots and pans made of brass, cooper and aluminium. People experiencing sleeping problems should only cook in stainless steel containers to avoid absorbing the above mentioned metals in their system, especially aluminium.

Many of us don't realize how hard our body is working to kill off the constant invasion of bacteria and viruses while also trying to compensate for the enormous physical strain, and rid itself of the harmful effect of alcohol, tobacco and excessive over eating.

I use the word excessive because I realize how important it is for a person who loves good food to eat, but over-eating places a terrible strain on the digestive system, heart, muscles and bones. If we cannot reduce the amount food we eat, we should at least help our system by eating a more fruit, which does not cause nearly as a great strain on the body as meat or fat. Try to look after your poor overworked body and in return it will reward you in more than one way.

Additional information on how to sleep better

1. One and a half hours before going to bed have a banana.
2. One hour before retiring eat some yoghurt. Place three tablespoons full of yoghurt in a bowl. Add two table spoons of oat bran, followed by two tablespoons of sesame seeds then two tablespoons of ground almonds finally add one teaspoon of honey. Mix well before eating.
3. Half an hour before retiring have half of a glass of skin milk with one magnesium tablet and a half a B6 tablet and one B12 tablet which should be chewed thoroughly.

If you wake up during the night have some apple juice with two valerian tablets.

The above mentioned ingredients are rich in Tryptophan which assists sleeping. Serotonin, derived from Tryptophan is a neurotransmitter triggers general feelings of happiness.

Yogurt is rich in lactobacillus which defends the body against harmful bacteria.

Oat bran is rich in vitamins and minerals and assists in the speedy removal of waste products.

Sesame seeds are a rich source of calcium, which is readily absorbed by the body to strengthen the bones and guard against limb or hip fractures.

Almonds help to fight cancer, they are rich in iron, essential for healthy blood cells. Vitamin B 12 is helpful against Alzheimer and depression. Magnesium supplements are useful to reduce blood pressure, diabetes, migraine, Asthma and angina.

Valerian is a natural sleep enhancer.

Don't drink coffee three hours before going to bed.

Don't do any exercise four hours before going to sleep.

Three hours before bed time avoid watching violent movies.

Drinking, smoking, and too much coffee will prevent you from sleeping well.

Don't do any boxing and avoid any activity may can cause frontal brain injury. Severe jarring of the brain incurred in blows to the head can cause depression mental problems and difficulty in sleeping.

Please note that the above mentioned food ingredients not only will help you to sleep better but it will make the elimination of waste products much faster in the morning.

Please note that people who are suffering from Narcolepsy, Sleep Apnoea or any unusual sleeping problems should not practice the sleep enhancing information mentioned above, or take any kind of sleeping pills. They should consult their GP for their sleep problems.

NON-BIOCHEMICAL SOLUTIONS FOR INSOMNIA

If the cause of insomnia is not related to food there are still a number of things that can be done to calm the mind and body so that sleep becomes natural.

- Meditate for at least 30 minutes before going to bed. You will often notice that during meditation you will fall asleep because you have achieved complete relaxation

- Practice your breathing exercise at home or at work. Try to take five minutes several times a day to practice body relaxation while sitting on a chair. First send your breath to your toes and relax, then send your breath to your feet and limbs, abdomen and chest, working your way up to the face and skull. Also, several times after 6pm clutch your hand and fingers together firmly for about five minutes about four times before going to bed.

- Walk for a half an hour every day, if this is not possible, then, at least do some exercise for ten minutes each session in the morning and afternoon. Avoid exercising right before going to bed.

- Do your pressure exercises every day. If it possible use a serrated wooden roller on your feet and hands for five minutes.

- Avoid watching films or reading stories with violent content two hours before bedtime. Instead listen to some music you like or read a book instead.

- Banish all feelings anger from your mind. When you feel excessive anger toward another person you are actually destroying yourself. Our situation is not the same as it was thousands of years ago when we needed our aggression response to fight and survive. These days the situation is often the opposite. We have to repress our anger and aggression to survive. I know this is easier said than done, but we have to tone down our aggressive responses so that we can function normally in modern society. As an alternative find expression for your natural aggression in work, sport and exercise.

- In bed relax and sing your favourite songs under your breath. It will make you drowsy and help you to fall asleep faster.

- Try to go to bed at the same time every night.

- Take a warm shower before going to bed.

- Before going to sleep think about yourself as calm person with tranquillity and peace of mind.

- Once you are in bed lay flat on your back, imagine that you are in a peaceful place where you were once were happy, perhaps one of your holidays. Have only pleasant and positive thoughts, perhaps about some lovely fishing trip, or a green meadow or a forest with deer running wild. When you feel that you are relaxed take a medium deep breath, hold it for the count of five then exhale slowly. Repeat this five times.

If you wake up at night tell yourself to relax, to be calm and go back to sleep in peace and quiet. If you have nightmares, don't worry. Nightmares are just dreams and are not real, with this attitude you can get used to nightmares. It is better to have nightmares and sleep than no nightmares and no sleep.

If you keep practicing meditation coupled with a healthy diet, then in time feeling completely relaxed will become second nature to you and sleep will become easy and natural for you.

SLEEP, THE MIND AND PATTERNS OF THINKING

According to doctors and psychiatrists the primary cause of insomnia is emotional disturbance. Much of this emotional disturbance comes from a general inability to properly deal with life's daily problems and has its roots in the early formation of our personality.

Many people are brainwashed in childhood by their parents or society into following a line of thinking or a code of behaviour which is unnatural and self-destructive.

Frequently, a child adopts a soul destroying instruction from an aggressive or incompetent mother or father only to find that later in their life this behaviour makes their life difficult. As time goes on the conflict within the person makes a heavy demand on their biological system in the form of constant tension. Tension impairs the body's ability to manufacture essential hormones and to absorb essential minerals and vitamins.

If we look around the world today, we see a great deal of conflict and violence. Violent tendencies often have their roots in personality traits inherited from fanatical or obsessive parents. The mind and body of a fanatical person is under a great strain. This strain is taxing and prematurely ages the body which in turn becomes prone to disease.

A fanatical or obsessive person might be able to sleep quite well, provided they can find an outlet for their frustration. However, when this is not possible, the unexpressed aggression is internalized making the person tense and nervous and causing difficulties in sleeping.

If all of us could follow a golden middle way this would save us a lot of misery. This middle way means being self-critical, understanding the consequences of our actions and realizing that extremes of behaviour are to be avoided and that moderation is required in everything.

The influence of parents, teachers and society is very strong during the early years of a child's growth when the mind is not yet logical or critical enough to distinguish between right and wrong. Bad codes of behaviour adopted in childhood are very difficult to change later in life especially if these senseless instructions are repeated by the parents.

At the other extreme, some of the parents teach that all immoral or aggressive thoughts are sinful. The feelings of guilt caused by these senseless teachings have caused a great deal of suffering among millions. In fact is there is no such thing as good or bad thoughts. There are only good or bad deeds. One does not help a fellow human being by only feeling sympathy for them. Conversely one does no harm to another just by having aggressive thoughts about them. It is deeds that count.

I am not advocating that one should cultivate aggressive thoughts, but simply tolerate them and not feel guilty about them.

If we stop taking annoying thoughts seriously, then in time they will cease to annoy us. People experiencing difficulties in sleeping should learn not to be angry with themselves for developing behaviour patterns which keep them tense and awake. Quarrels or anger directed against oneself only puts oil on the fire.

It is essential to avoid self-inflicted emotion which will cause turmoil in a person, especially at night. All emotion is a response to external events. It is up to us how we react to external stimulus. You are in control of your emotions they are not in control of you. Emotional responses are often disproportionate to the actual event which caused them. It is important to think rationally and have a sense of perspective when thinking and not sink into a self-created whirlpool of emotional turmoil. Whenever one feels that one would like to change their behaviour pattern, it should be done slowly and peacefully.

Try talking to yourself before falling asleep using positive affirmations. For example recite the following:

- I will relax deeply relax.
- I will have peace and quiet in my mind.
- I will sleep deeply and peacefully without nightmares.
- I will cease to practice damaging behaviour patterns which make me unable to sleep.
- I will follow the golden middle way of behaviour, which will give me calmness and tranquillity.
- I will avoid agitating my mind unnecessarily and will calm myself by exhaling bad thoughts with each breath.

As I say these things I feel a sense of serenity and tranquillity coming over me.

I am looking forward to the day when I will stop taking things too seriously during my work or at home and feel relaxed and calm in both places.

Practice meditation and deep breathing exercises.

Seek to discard dependency on drugs such as sleeping pills. They don't work on the long run anyway.

Using these techniques we take control of our life and our emotions.

People who are prone to high tension, ambitious or subject to persecution from parents and teachers, are particularly at risk of suffering high blood pressure, stress, heart attacks not to mention sleeping disorders.

It is quite understandable for us to feel anger toward parents or teachers who have caused us anguish by teaching us the wrong things but let's not forget that they themselves were probably helpless pawns in the hands of their own parents and teachers who did the same.

It is our duty not only to look after our body but our mind as well, to calm ourselves in difficult or even in hopeless situations. We must think of ourselves as valuable and banish thoughts of low self-esteem and guilt. Everyone deserves to sleep.

Have confidence in the relaxation methods you have learned and the future will bring you more peace and tranquillity and better all-round health.

If you really want to be a good human being then once you have looked after yourself, try helping other people as well. We are social animals. The sense of self-esteem gained by helping others will make you happy and help your sleep better.

SECTION 6. ACUPRESSURE, HEALING IN YOUR HANDS

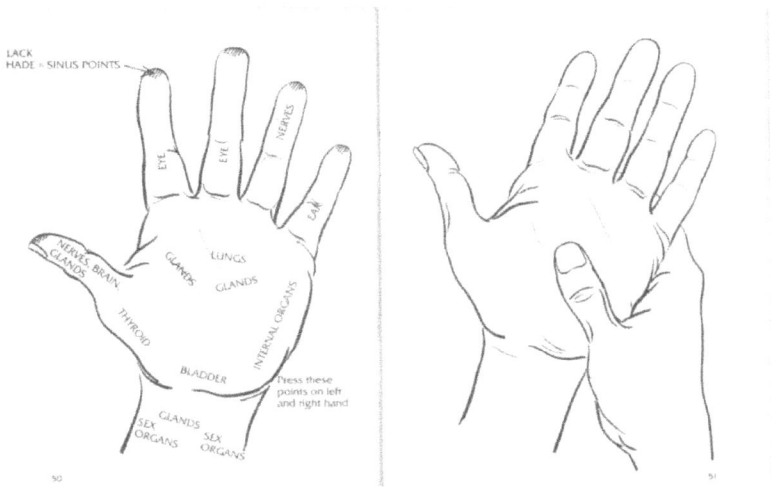

Figure 2. Healing pressure technique

In the previous chapters we have discovered that meditation is a way to not only to improve our mental and physical health, but also to give new meaning to our lives.

Now I would like to introduce another method of healing. The first one is the healing pressure technique, the second is breathing.

First we shall discuss the pressure technique. This consists of applying mild pressure to various parts of the palm of the hand.

The origin of this ancient technique is lost in antiquity. It is the product of countless years of observation by healers in India called Rishis and Sages, who treated people in ancient times suffering from a variety of physical and mental problems. Written records of this technique date back some 2.500 years, unfortunately most of the written records have been destroyed through war and fire.

One branch of the body pressure technique was taken and developed further in China where it became known as acupuncture.

The advantage of the pressure technique over acupuncture is that you don't need a qualified practitioner to insert needles into your body you can apply the technique yourself.

In the pressure technique, as in acupuncture one of the basic goals is to restore the electrical balance of the body. Once the proper balance is restored, the healing process starts.

HOW TO APPLY PRESSURE

You need to use your thumb as a pressure instrument. For example, apply pressure to the palm of your hand by moving the thumb of your other hand over the top of your palm in a horizontal movement supported by the rest of your fingers on the side of your hand.

To start press about one inch below the palm, near where your pulse can be felt on your wrist. Do not press too hard, just enough to feel it. Follow the horizontal line and work your way up line by line, until you covered the whole surface of the palm, then start on your fingers. Work your thumb up from the base of each finger to the very top. Press all points including the finger nails, then go back to the center of the palm, where the thumb should press down vertically in a radius of two inches, or five centimetres. The reason is that the center of the palm of each hand is connected to the glands of your body. By pressing these points we send electrical stimulation to the glands and restore their functions.

The duration of each pressing action should be approximately five to ten seconds. It should take approximately five minutes including the fingers to cover one hand.

Now we come to an important point. During our routine pressing, you may occasionally feel pain. When you do, stop for a moment. Pain indicates a particular point on our palm or finger which is connected to a part of our body where sickness or trouble lies. Stay on the trouble spot and press again for two solid minutes. If you find that the pain persists, repeat the process on the same point, three times a day, one or two minutes at a time until the pain disappears.

The technique can also be applied to the soles of the feet. If you find it difficult to do the pressure technique on the feet get yourselves a wooden rolling pin with serrated edges and roll your soles on it for five minutes per foot.

Do not expect any instant cures. However, if you practice your pressure technique for five minutes on each hand and foot, within a few weeks you should see the positive difference in your general health. The benefits of the pressure technique are twofold:

- It will help you to lose weight if you are overweight.
- It will improve your digestion.

Note: People suffering from cancer or women who are pregnant, should not use pressure technique.

WHERE TO APPLY PRESSURE

- If you have a pain in the breast, press the center of the back of your palm. If you feel pain when you press, then instead of the normal five seconds, press for two minutes twice daily. Please note, all pressing should be done in a pumping fashion up and down. Pressure technique can be applied to other parts of the body besides the palm and feet to treat specific problems:

- For chest pain, press the center of the outside arm between the palm and the elbow.

- For headache press the inner part of the thumb on both the left and right hands, from the top of the thumb to the base, and practice deep breathing.

- To treat problems associated with your back, press the back of your palm between the thumb and the first finger. If you feel any pain at all keep pressing for the usual two minutes twice a day.

- If you suffer from influenza or sinus problems, use your thumb to press the base of your nose for two to three minutes on the left side, then for the same of time on the right side. Also press the center point of your forehead just under the hair line and the center of your forehead between your eyebrows.

- For urinary problems press all points on both left and right wrists and drink six glasses of water per day to clean out toxins from the body. Drinking water will also help the kidneys to function better.

SECTION 7. CANCER

THE CAUSES OF CANCER

Cancer can be hereditary e.g. hereditary breast cancer; Cancer can be caused by external factors such as radiation or exposure to chemicals, for example, exposure to asbestos dust and excessive sun tanning.

Here we concentrate on cancer caused by bad lifestyle and dietary habits. That is, things we can control.

Cancer does not happen overnight. Cancer is the end product of continuous abuse and neglect of our bodies over many years. Here is a list of self-inflicted practices which over time can cause cancer:

Bowel cancer can be caused by eating refined food, e.g. white flour, white rice, sugar. Please note that sugar should be considered a poison, especially refined sugar. Cancer cells thrive on sugar and cannot survive without it. Bowel cancer can also be caused by excessive consumption of alcohol.

Eating or drinking hot food for many years can cause stomach cancer. Stomach cancer is also prevalent In Japan where people have a high percentage of salt in their diet.

There is a direct link between smoking and lung cancer.

Cancer of the uterus and cervix can be caused by unhygienic sexual practices. Men should always wash before intercourse and women should always wash after.

Decades of medical research have shown that eating various nuts, fruit and vegetable consumption will sharply reduce the possibility of cancer, heart attack and stroke as well as eye problems, which might lead to blindness.

On the other hand excessive consumption of refined food, meat, especially beef and pork, can not only cause cancer, but contribute to high blood pressure, arthritis and glaucoma.

According to medical research the body only needs 60 grams of protein daily. If you eat more than this the body must work hard to process it and consequently have less energy for healing purposes.

WHY CANCER

The body is working day and night to replace cells, detoxify the blood and produce enzymes for digestion. The liver, kidneys, lymph glands and spleen are responsible for this process. If the body is subjected to overload, because of an unhealthy diet, detoxification regeneration of new cells is retarded. The body gets poisoned and cancerous tumours develop. Warning signs include loss of weight headache, fever and pain.

In the previous chapter it was pointed out, that with the aid of meditation, the right diet and breathing exercises, cancer is unlikely to develop.

Cancer is curable in its early stages provided the person is willing to change their lifestyle and diet.

In general vegetarians are less likely to get cancer however vegetarians often have low cholesterol which is another cause of cancer. For this reason it is important that vegetarians include enough unsaturated fat in their diet.

Even when you have cancer all is not lost as you can heal yourself, positive thinking essential.

I would like to emphasize that that modern medicine is essential, and the above information is only to be used in addition to conventional medicine.

THE MAGIC OF FLAXSEED OIL

Dr. Johanna Budwig worked for many years to find a fatty acid that will help the body to absorb vitamins, as well as act as an anti-cancer agent. Her work was carried on by Udo Eramus.

As a result of years of research she found a substance which did just that, Flaxseed oil.

Flaxseed oil is a rich source of Omega 3 and is a very important product against Cancer, diabetes, hypertension, high blood pressure, and a great number of other ailments.

As well as fighting cancer, Flaxseed oil does the following:

- Reduces symptoms of diabetes.
- Promotes proper liver function
- Reduces hypertension
- Vital for brain function and helps people with mental illness
- A useful fibre and helps the prostate.
- Reduces blood pressure and cholesterol
- Good against arthritis
- Fights anaemia
- Helps back pain
- Reduces cataracts
- Helps male impotence
- Fights Parkinson's disease
- Reduces Psoriasis

- Eases stomach problems
- Eases constipation
- Improves vision and hearing
- Prevents kidney degeneration
- Helps the immune system
- Reduce stomach acid
- Reduces chronic fatigue
- Eases symptoms of menopause.

Flaxseed oil is particularly helpful as an anti-tumor agent in cases of colon cancer

HOW TO TAKE FLAXSEED OIL

Take two full soup spoons of flaxseed oil with carrot juice daily.

Once a day take vitamin E.

After using flaxseed oil for ten months add one spoonful of Udos oil to your regime.

Udos oil contains various vitamins and minerals not contained in flaxseed oil. Flaxseed oil and Udos oil can be purchased in health stores. For people who can't tolerate swallowing oils it is also available in linseeds.

BREAST CANCER

Japan is a first world country with a very low incidence of breast cancer. There is a direct link between the low incidence of breast cancer and the eating habits of the Japanese nation. Researchers have found that a diet rich in fruit, vegetables, and fresh fish, is largely responsible for the absence of breast cancer in Japanese women. The relatively small number of diagnosed breast cancers occurred mainly in the more affluent classes who were able to afford more beef in their diet. This disease did not affect the less wealthy section of the female population whose traditional food intake consists of fruit, fish and vegetables. Generally speaking Japanese women are healthier than Japanese men. Perhaps a reason for this is that it is bad manners for Japanese women to drink and smoke.

American researchers found, that when Japanese women moved to the USA they developed the same proportion of breast cancer as American women.

So in order reduce the possibility of cancer, one should follow the Japanese eating habits.

A note for mothers: If possible breast feed your baby. This will reduce the chance of your child getting breast cancer later on in life.

Ask your GP to check your breasts for abnormal growths at least twice a year.

COLON AND BOWEL CANCER

Colon cancer can be caused by eating junk food for a long time and a lack of roughage in people's diet. That is, not enough fruit and vegetables. Please note that cholesterol is re-absorbed by the body in the intestines unless roughage is present.

Chronic constipation also contributes to colon cancer. The longer waste products stay in the colon, the more likelihood of developing colon cancer. For the dangerous microbes not to multiply in the colon, it is essential that one should eliminate waste products at least twice a day.

It is important that waste is removed from the colon regularly. We need to eat foods that keep us regular. Tomatoes are a good source of roughage and help the colon to move waste products faster. The lactobacilli in yoghurt will kill all other harmful bacteria in the stomach and the intestine.

If a child is not breast fed for at least four months, then the small intestine can become porous and damaged, and it will let food particles into the blood stream without proper digestion. The imperfectly digested food particles instead of being fully utilized by the body as fuel can attack the white and red blood cells causing havoc and as a result you feel sick in more ways than one.

Drinking six glasses of water each day can decrease the risk of colon cancer.

Damage to the small intestine can also occur as a result of viral infection.

THE ANTI-CANCER DIET

If the body is supported by the right diet then the chance of developing cancer is sharply reduced.

Firstly here is a list of foods not to eat. Unhealthy foods which contain cacogenic agents include:

Peanuts, beer, sugar, pickled vegetables, barbecued meat, deep fried potato chips and margarine.

One should completely cut out sugar as cancer can't survive without sugar.

Do not drink more than one cup of coffee or tea per day.

Avoid eating animal fats including all oils with the exception of virgin olive oil.

While on an anti-cancer diet one should not drink milk, all dairy products create mucus in the body on which cancer thrives. A little butter in your diet is acceptable.

For minerals take Selenium, Magnesium, Calcium and Iron.

Anti-carcinogenic agents are vitamins, anti-oxidants, flaxseed oil, fish oil, apricot kernels, ginseng, Echinacea, apples, pears, nuts, beans, seeds, cherries, nectarines, cabbage, Brussels sprouts, carrots, tomatoes, onion, papaya, turnips, bee pollen, avocado, beans, cabbage, garlic, mangos, onions, dark grapes and lemon juice. Lemon juice is a particularly important as an anti-cancer agent. Use the juice of one lemon mixed with some carrot juice three times daily. Lemon juice is an excellent cancer fighting agent and will also reduce high blood pressure.

Additional cancer fighting agents are Echinacea, Grass powder, Omega 3 fish oil, Green tea and Pau d'Arco tea.

Have a glass of wheat grass juice daily.

Garlic will kill cancer cells. Eat raw garlic or a garlic tablet daily.

In the case of advanced cancer one should use seven table spoons of flaxseed oil daily mixed with carrot juice, a month later five spoonful's of flaxseed oil and each month later one spoonful less.

Flaxseed oil will increase oxidation improving sharply the body's intake of oxygen. Various germs such as Candida cannot tolerate high oxygen levels in the body.

Note that excessive use of antibiotics or cortisone can cause cancer.

Meditate at least two hours daily. While you meditate use your imagination and concentrate on the area where you have cancer and visualize billions of T cells surrounding the disease with an iron ring and tearing the cancerous cells apart.

Another good agent for fighting cancer is Cinnamon. Once a day take one teaspoon of cinnamon powder add some warm water so it dissolves properly and drink it in one gulp with a half of cup of carrot juice.

In addition take two tablets of inner health daily after food. Please note that the health oils and the inner health tablets must be kept in the refrigerator at all times.

Ask your GP to send you for a blood allergy test. You may be allergic to certain food products which will contribute to your sickness.

Here is a summarized list of things to include in the anti-cancer diet:

- Cut down or eliminate alcohol.
- Reduce the intake of coffee and tea.
- Take one folic acid tablet after meals daily and two Brazil nuts.
- Stay away from canned food.
- Drink six glasses of purified water or fruit juice daily.
- Cut out the consumption of red meat completely.
- Eat a raw carrot every second day.
- Eat four eggs a week, or more without the egg yolks.
- Reduce the amount of animal fat in your diet.
- Eat well washed fruit and vegetables, one piece of raw garlic (which kills cancer cells) and a handful of almonds or walnuts to avoid eye problems.
- Reduce your intake of salt but don't cut it out completely as it

is essential to have some salt in your diet. If you do take salt, it should be Iodized salt to prevent Goitre.

- Eliminate the intake of refined sugar and white bread.

- Use whole meal flour in baking.

- Three times a week take some multi vitamin tablets including Zinc and Vitamin C. With your evening meal have a half of lemon juice with mixed with some apple juice.

- Stay away from hot food and cold drinks.

- Eat slowly and chew your food well before swallowing it.

- Take two table spoons of Flaxseed or Udo's oil with four spoons of yoghurt and a mashed banana every second day.

- Use only virgin olive oil, do not use margarine.

- Don't eat when not hungry.

- Drink a glass of lukewarm water every morning if constipated.

- Have the juice of half a lemon mixed with some apple juice every day.

- Don't drink water kept or sold in plastic bottles

LIFESTYLE CHANGES TO AVOID CANCER

- Sleep as much as possible when you are sick
- Don't smoke
- Clean your air conditioning filter once a month
- Exercise at least 20 minutes daily

- Practice meditation daily
- Walk or swim whenever possible.
- Do deep breathing exercises twice a day for five minutes at a time.
- Whenever possible use an old fashioned phone rather than your mobile or cordless phone, as according to a number of scientists mobile phones can cause brain damage
- Avoid all non-essential drugs, hair dyes, perfumes, shaving lotions and toothpaste
- Don't use aluminium pots for cooking.
- Watch as many comedy videos as possible. Laughter is a wonderful anti-cancer agent.

ADVANCED CANCER

According to research it is possible to reverse cancer if not too far advanced. Even in advanced stages the symptoms of cancer can be alleviated considerably if one follows strict guide lines.

- Drink a glass of warm purified water twice daily.
- For the first seven days drink only freshly squeezed fruit or vegetable juices and one glasses of carrot juice.

After that you can introduce vegetables such as beetroot, broccoli, lentils, paw- paw, asparagus, brown rice, millet, buck wheat and beans.

For breakfast you can have soya, tofu, and salads, rolled oats, mashed bananas and apples. For nuts, in the early part of the diet eat only ground almonds

After two months you can add a small amount of well boiled chicken, turkey, and some fish. After six months you can halve the intake of flaxseed oil and add instead Udos oil, once a day.

SECTION 8. PROSTATE PROBLEMS

We live in the age of pills. There are pills to fight infectious diseases, pills to reduce high blood pressure, pills for sleeping, pills for staying awake, pain killers, vitamins the list goes on.

However, at present there is no pill to stop the degeneration of the prostate.

Maybe there will be in the future. Meanwhile if you want to save yourself a lot of misery and suffering then please take advantage of the information given below.

The prostate gland is only present in males. It is approximately the size of a walnut. Its main function is to secrete semen which carries sperm cells out of the body. The gland is situated partly under the bladder and the urinary tract. The urethra is a tube which empties urine coming from the bladder.

As men grow older the prostate gland becomes larger. In many cases it will press upon the bladder and the Urethral tube, reducing or sometimes cutting the flow of urine from the bladder. If this happens, then an operation is needed to save the person's life. The first indication of a prostate problem is that one has to go the toilet four to six times during the night to relieve oneself. Other symptoms are a burning sensation in the penis, blood in the urine and pain in the rectum.

In order to postpone, or possibly eliminate the deterioration of the prostate and the bladder, we should start a set of simple exercises. These exercises will increase the size and capacity of the bladder and the prostate gland will shrink in size. Here are the exercises:

- Contract your muscles in your anus approximately 50 times while sitting on a chair, the same way as you would contract your arm muscles. To be exact contract and release, contract and release.

- When you urinate, stop the flow of urine for a second, by contracting the muscles in your penis, then resume urinating. Do this every time when urinating but not when sitting on the toilet. You will notice that after a while this exercise will strengthen the muscles in your penis. It will also reduce the effect of impotentence. If you keep on doing this for weeks, gradually the flow of urine will become stronger and easier and at the same time it will strengthen your prostate. This exercise will keep your prostate small and more muscular, so in time you will have no trouble sleeping through the night without going to the toilet.

- Put both of your hands together firmly on the lower part of your stomach when on the toilet and then massage your stomach gently in a circular fashion. Do that about a hundred times or more. You will feel a sensation going through your penis, which is a similar sensation to the one when a doctor is massaging your prostate in order to clear an obstruction. Please note that this exercise is not suitable for people who had, or in the near future will have an abdominal operation.

- Push your whole body including your head and body back and forth toward to the rear of the toilet cistern about a hundred times or more.

- Lift your head then push it with a jerking movement to the right, then to the left. Do this a hundred times or more.

- Put both your right and left palms on your upper forehead and massage your forehead and chin vigorously for about a hundred times in a circular fashion.

You will find that exercises five and six will make you sneeze, this is normal.

All these exercises will promote the removal of waste products from the intestines which is a breeding ground for infection and disease. Exercise number four will in time also reduce pain in your spine, as well as strengthen your back.

I would like to emphasize, that the 'health exercises' will not only benefit men, but women as well whose bladder function will improve and who will notice that after a few months their body will become trimmer, the tone of their skin smother and the wrinkles on their face will be reduced. Exercises three, four and five will also be beneficial for women who have bladder problems

Another beneficial side effect of the above mentioned exercises is that it will gently massage all of your other internal organs like your liver, kidney, pancreas and various glands and prevent their degeneration.

People who already have cancer of the Prostate, or are about to have an operation should **NOT** and I say again **NOT** do any of the physical exercises, however the dietary information as described previously should be followed.

The exercises will save you a great deal of energy in digestion, so the body will be able to concentrate on healing itself and reduce the possibility of heart attacks , strokes, cancer and Alzheimer's.

PROSTATE PROBLEMS AND DIET

One of the reasons for prostate problems is the lack of fruit and vegetables in the diet Fruit and vegetables provide a source of roughage which in turn helps the colon to get rid the waste products. Each time men have a motion, the prostate is slightly massaged and this is exactly what the prostate needs, to be massaged in order not to degenerate.

Garlic is especially good for maintaining a healthy prostate as well as for general health as mentioned in the food section of this book. Other foods which promote prostate health are vegetables such as carrots, onion, peas and cabbage lentils, which contain a lot of iron.

Tomatoes are one of the best antioxidants and reduce the possibility of prostate cancer.

The above mentioned exercises and diet will not only help your prostate, but will reduce the possibility of getting colon cancer, help your bladder stay healthy, it will gently massage of all your other vital organs such as your liver, kidneys, and pancreas as well.

All of the mentioned exercises and dietary suggestions will also benefit women who are incontinent.

The above mentioned exercises will not only prevent prostate problems, but at the same time will exercise most of your muscles and reduce arthritis and back pain.

All medical health experts agree that in order to reduce the possibility of strokes, heart attacks, and mental tension, exercise is essential.

In fact when you do the above mentioned muscular movements, you are exercising. At the same time you are rapidly getting rid of your accumulated waste products, which if they stay more than three days in your intestines, could become the breeding ground for carcinogenic material, which in time could cause cancer.

It might take a week or two before your body will properly react to the health exercise. After a while you will notice that you will go to the toilet two or three times a day, especially if you increase fruit, nuts and vegetables in your diet.

As a rule most people spend ten to fifteen minutes on the toilet waiting for their sluggish body to react. Start the day by drinking a glass of warm water and walk a few minutes before going to the toilet. When you are sitting on the toilet you should start your prostate exercises as described above.

Using the above information spend your time rather doing your health exercises at least five minutes each time when you go to the toilet. In the long run it will re- vitalize your body and make you healthier.

If you wish you can ask your doctor for an opinion or follow the same exercise I do of your own free will. I would like to point out that the above exercises gave me a one hundred per cent result.

IMPORTANCE OF THE GLANDS

Our glands play a very important role in keeping us healthy. The pituitary controls the adrenal thyroid and the sex glands. The previous exercises associated with the prostate exercises will help to keep all the glands healthy both for men and women.

SECTION 9. SEX

THE SEXUAL NEEDS OF WOMEN

Throughout the ages the idea that women have sexual needs and desires has been the subject of scorn and ridicule by society.

The reasons for their deprivation were many.

To start with the Catholic Church looked upon sex as a necessary evil. Sex was necessary for procreation only and it was sinful to enjoy it. It was responsible for creating a guilt complex among its followers of things associated with the body and with sex.

The feeling of guilt made the full enjoyment of sex difficult if not impossible.

In the east women did not fare much better as they were considered nothing more than objects created to satisfy men.

Going back in the past as far as ancient times the knowledge of how to satisfy women sexually was known to but a few.

In modern time thanks to less dogmatic thinking and more open discussion knowledge about women's needs is now gradually being recognized.

Women as a rule respond to sexual stimulation much slower than men and require a certain degree of foreplay. Foreplay includes kissing as well as fondling of their breasts and other body parts including their clitoris so they can then proceed to orgasm.

ADVICE FOR MEN

If you care about your wife or girlfriend, then follow some

suggestions.

Be compassionate to her, help her with domestic chores, tell her that you love her, tell her how lovely she looks and take her out at least twice a week to a restaurant or some entertainment.

When she is sick, give her help and sympathy.

Treat her as friend as well rather than a sex object.

Ask her about her desires, her problems and hopes.

When making love, don't forget about foreplay. Ask her what variations she would like to have in sex. When you start making love to her, do it slowly in a relaxed way so you don't get too excited too quickly. When you see that she is excited enough then start to concentrate on your pleasure only so both of you can have an orgasm together.

ERECTILE DYSFUNCTION

Through the centuries middle aged men considered their virility a very important asset. To have a proper erection and perform sexually is important for a man's self-confidence.

As men age, many will find that their erection is not as hard as it used to be and at times their erection is not sufficient to have sexual intercourse . When this happens it causes a great deal of anguish in men, as well as to their wives or partners.

The cause for the lack of erection can be psychological as well biological.

As we all know heart attacks are often the result of arteries getting clogged with a fatty substance called Cholesterol. The same fatty material will eventually restrict the flow of blood through the penis and results in a lack of proper erection.

Other reasons for sexual difficulties are as follows:

High blood pressure, diabetes, prostate problems, smoking, excessive drinking, stress, anger toward your sexual partner, depression and feelings of guilt or being too eager to please your partner.

So in order to heal yourself, please follow some guidelines.

- Reduce the amount of all fats except perhaps a little butter.
- Stop smoking. Smoking will not only severely damage your blood vessels but it will also reduce your ability to have sex. The same damage is done by excessive alcohol.
- Follow the previously mentioned dietary guidelines.
- Take one Ginkgo tablet daily after breakfast.
- Eat one banana every day.
- Ask your GP for a prescription of Testosterone gel.
- Do your prostate exercises as described previously.
- Meditate when you have a chance to reduce tension.
- Go for a long walk whenever possible, or do some exercise at home.
- Discuss your problem with your partner.
- Visit your GP and ask for an examination. However the following products will stimulate sexual desire to some extent. Five hours before sex have some Vitamin E and ZINC. Also, two tablespoonful's of Lecithin Granules with a glass of water one hour before sex.
- Take Flaxseed oil every day as well ginseng and ginkgo tablet one hour before sex.

- Add one piece of raw garlic to your diet.

If you can manage a half an erection that will be enough to have sex provided you do it from the rear and put a small amount of moisturizer on the penis.

TESTOSTERONE, OESTROGEN, SEROTONIN, L-DOPA

Serotonin is manufactured in the brain from amino acids with the help of vitamin B6, B12 and folic acid. Serotonin is a very important product which has many functions. It is essential for sleep and to avoid depression.

Some men who are low in serotonin will at times experience confusion and depression after sex. In that case eating a whole banana will restore the much needed serotonin and after a short while the confusion will disappear.

Depressions and mood disorders are not only caused by traumas based on one's past unpleasant experiences, but may also be caused by nutrient deficiencies. A good diet and some vitamins will reverse the problem.

Food allergies can also cause depression.

If you are suffering from depression avoid caffeine containing drinks and food additives.

The right amount of L-dopa, a brain chemical, will not only guard you from depression, but it is also essential for satisfactory sex.

The lack of testosterone can be a curse and causes a great deal of anguish among millions of men who are yearning for good sexual satisfaction.

Viagra for this problem is not a solution, as it will only work if one has a strong sexual desire.

Unfortunately a great deal of Viagra on the market is useless, as it is not genuine. It is safer to buy Cialis.

Note that if one is having macular degeneration then it is advisable to stay away from Viagra, Cialis and any sort of a drug which contains cortisone.

At present there are a number of drug companies who are working to create a drug which will cause desire and a hard erection at the same time.

Research scientist in USA found that excessive amounts of testosterone are often responsible for rape and increased violence.

In the USA many prisoners have this problem. In general men who are responsible for domestic violence have more testosterone in their blood. In the USA there are eight times more male prisoners than women, the number of murders committed by males is much higher than of women.

Testosterone is the main reason that men are far more aggressive than women. Excessive amounts of testosterone will damage the immune system. Men with a vast amount of testosterone are less able to manufacture antibodies then women. As a result men will find it more difficult to fight cancer and resist infection. The rate of suicide among young men with extra large amount of testosterone is three times higher than young women. The mortality rate among men living alone is twice as high as for spinsters. Scientist found that women are less likely to get heart attacks then men because the oestrogen in their blood is protecting their heart.

As a rule, women live ten years longer than men and the hormonal differences between the sexes may be the reason for this.

SECTION 10. SUGGESTIONS FOR HEALTHY MEALS

BREAKFAST

The following is a breakdown of the ultimate breakfast:

- Have three tablespoons of plain yoghurt.
- A half or a whole finely chopped apple, or pear. Peel the skin before eating
- Two table spoons of washed, desiccated coconuts and two pieces of well washed apricots.
- Two Brazil nuts.
- One tablespoon of chopped almonds and one tablespoon of walnuts.
- One table spoon of sesame seeds
- Dark grapes
- Two pieces of seedless prunes
- One cup of herbal tea, half tea, half apple juice.

All fruit should be chopped, please note that all dried fruits should be well washed with warm water to remove traces of fungus.

WHY IS THIS GOOD FOR YOU?

Yoghurt: Yoghurt is a friendly bacillus which will assist digestion.

The lactobacilli in yoghurt will kill all other harmful bacteria in the stomach and in the intestine. Yoghurt with lactobacilli in it has many useful roles in the body including better digestion, reducing bowel symptoms; it also helps to absorb useful minerals, such as magnesium and calcium. It also kills harmful bacteria.

If you are on antibiotics, then take daily lactobacilli tablets to replace your internal flora.

Apples: Improves lung capacity.

Apricots: Fight cancer, control blood pressure, promote good vision, protects against Alzheimer and slow the aging process.

Dates: Rich in minerals and vitamins.

Prunes: Promote good digestion and bowel movement.

Brazil nuts: The richest source of selenium, a great anti-oxidant and essential to keep the brain healthy.

Almonds and walnuts: Lower cholesterol, fight cancer, helps memory retention. Good for the heart.

Sesame seeds: The richest source of calcium, needed in the body to prevent bone breakage.

Coconuts: Rich in essential minerals

All the above mentioned food products will prevent constipation and reduce the risk of colon cancer.

Please note that fruit and the above mentioned products should be eaten on an empty stomach and not be mixed with other foods.

It only takes one hour to digest this breakfast, after which, if you need a snack, you can have some toasted rye bread with a small amount of butter, never eat margarine.

LUNCH

For lunch eat sardines with a slice of rye bread, or cheese and avocado, or assorted vegetables and some yoghurt.

DINNER

At dinner eat a lot of vegetables, tomatoes with a little poultry. Do not eat red or any other type of meat.

Discontinue eating all margarines or oils except virgin olive oil. A little butter is OK.

In the long run this diet will improve your general health and give your body a chance to heal itself.

SECTION 11. HEART DISEASE AND HIGH BLOOD PRESSURE

The heart beats close to a hundred thousand times a day pumping five litres of blood per minute around your body, which adds up seven thousand litres in over 24 hours.

When the blood starts its journey, it is saturated with oxygen which flows from the left side to the aorta then through the arteries to every cell in the body giving them vital oxygen and various nutrients. As the blood moves waste is removed and with the aid of the lungs fresh oxygen is supplied.

The heart fundamentally has three major components; the muscles, the valves and its nervous system. If one of those is damaged, it can endanger life.

The main killer is coronary artery disease which can reduce the flow of blood to the heart muscle. The other problem affecting the heart is a fatty deposit in the inner lining of the coronary arteries which can affect the heart muscle, but not the rest of the heart.

If the flow of blood is sharply reduced because of blockage and damage to inner walls then less blood reaches the muscles and Angina develops a very painful and dangerous condition.

Heart valves can also be damaged by rheumatic disease which usually starts after a bacterial infection.

The heart's nervous system is regulated by a rhythm associated with an electric, chemical, and muscular time keeping mechanism, if this system breaks down a pace maker must be installed.

One could write hundreds of pages on various factors affecting the heart. I am not qualified to do that. However, I firmly believe that a healthy life style can prevent much of the miseries associated with heart disease.

To start with smoking and heavy alcohol consumption will do damage to the heart, as well as being overweight and a sedentary life style. Daily exercise is a must. Modern life is full of stress, so one should compensate by relaxing meditation.

A lot of people in rich countries have some blockage in their arteries. The main reason is high levels of cholesterol. Research scientists found that health problems are less prevalent in Japan then in most other countries due to their diet low in fat and rich in fruit and vegetables, as well the heavy consumption of fish.

Heart problems are caused by high blood pressure, high level of cholesterol in the blood, smoking, and diabetes, enlargement of the left ventricle, depression, obesity and marital disharmony (Broken Heart).

High blood pressure, also known as hypertension is a silent killer. High blood pressure can manifest itself in the following ways:

- irregular heartbeat
- tiredness
- memory lapses
- nose bleeds
- impotence
- dizziness
- headaches
- bowel and bladder problems
- stomach acid
- allergies
- chest pain

- bad dreams and difficulty falling asleep
- short temper
- premenstrual symptoms

As a rule, blood pressure is never constant; it is subject to change according to a person's physical condition and state of mind. However, a lifetime of wrong eating and drinking habits will definitely clog up the main arteries forcing the heart to pump harder until a constant state of high blood pressure arises.

The ideal blood pressure is 120 over 80. This figure is subject to change, especially if a person is over 60 years old.

Constant high blood pressure can cause heart attacks, strokes, kidney damage, as well as eye and brain damage.

High blood pressure makes the heart work harder than it should and in the long run can endanger one's life.

Anyone concerned about blood pressure should have their blood pressure checked at least twice a year by a GP.

High blood pressure can be inherited but with the right diet and exercise we can reduce its damaging effects.

There are various drugs to treat heart trouble, such as Digitalis extract, cardiac glycosides, or beta blockers. There are also drugs to dissolve blood clots. See your GP for further information.

WHAT CAN BE DONE

After breakfast, have one grape seed capsule. Grape seed helps to keep blood pressure normal. Grape seed capsules are available in health food stores. Also, include a piece of raw garlic in your morning meal.

Reduce your intake of salt. There is a direct correlation between salt and high blood pressure.

Sharply reduce the intake of alcohol, stop smoking, stay away from all refined foods such as white flour, white sugar, margarine and all saturated fats such as lard and oils with the exception of virgin olive oil, some butter is OK. Have pure fruit or vegetable juices, do not drink soft drinks and do not eat junk food.

Do not drink more than one cup of coffee or tea per day.

Useful vitamins for reducing blood pressure are: vitamins A, C, D, Calcium and Magnesium (500 mg each) and Potassium. One of the most important vitamins is vitamin E which will reduce the possibility of strokes.

Foods which will reduce blood pressure are: Brazil nuts (2 pieces per day), cheddar cheese, almonds, sardines, spinach, yoghurt, skim milk, coconut, radish, carrots, beans, cucumber, garlic, cabbage, tomatoes, melon, orange, banana, lemon juice mixed with a half a glass of fruit juice and apple.

Foods which contain fibre or anti-oxidants will reduce blood pressure. These will improve blood circulation, reduce heart attacks and strokes and will balance sugar levels. Bananas can reduce the incidence of strokes. Bananas reduce the excessive amount of stomach acid and helps sleep. They will calm the nerves it will help to get rid of waste products. Bananas are also helpful against depression. They will stimulate the production of red blood cells and can help people to give up smoking. Bananas are high in vitamins such as B6, B12, potassium, magnesium, Vitamin E, B, C and Gingko. Other useful foods which will lower blood pressure are: Echinacea, hawthorn and lemon juice.

Flaxseed oil, fish oil will also help reduce blood pressure (see chapter on Cancer/The magic of Flaxseed oil). Ginkgo tablets are also helpful.

Reduce the consumption of processed or smoked chicken, don't eat beef or pork. If you buy peas, buy frozen peas not canned.

Take some folic acid tablets as well as magnesium, and calcium.

Maintain a healthy weight. Excess weight places a heavy burden on the heart and decreases life expectancy.

Prescription drugs are available to bring down high blood pressure. Ask your GP for these.

Tranquilizers and sedatives will not help keep your blood pressure down but half an hour daily meditation will help a lot.

In order to keep blood pressure low we need to try to reduce stress and anxiety. To do this we must exercise. Walking, dancing and swimming are good exercises.

Depression and stress can also contribute to high blood pressure as they create cortisone which will raise blood pressure and attack the eyes and brain. For example when we are under pressure in a job, or even in heavy traffic our blood pressure goes up.

Meditate, walk or exercise at least a half an hour daily, this will reduce stress. Avoid feelings of anger, hatred, and vengeance. Be forgiving to yourself and others.

Practice deep breathing five or ten minutes daily.

In order to control our blood pressure we should let our rational brain control our aggressive responses. Uncontrolled anger can end in violence giving rise to symptoms of high blood pressure, depression, panic attacks, difficulty of concentrating, loss of memory, migraine head attacks, allergies, phobias and back ache.

Negative experiences in everyday life can create tension and emotional upset.

The family can upset us e.g. the lack of love from a child, wife or husband. External difficulties upset us e.g. financial problems, difficult working conditions, harsh bosses, over-work, disputes with neighbours. Often these problems escalate and become uncontrollable. When a person becomes obsessive, fanatical and loses control then logic reason and common sense disappears.

The world has always been a very violent place. In order to reduce our stress we should not take things to seriously.

HOW TO RECOGNIZE A HEART ATTACK

How do you know if you are having a heart attack?

Warning signs of heart attacks are intense pain in the left arm and chest as well as excessive sweating. You will also experience excessive tiredness, shortness of breath, feeling cold in the arm, tightening of the chest, neck and jaw.

How do you know if someone is having a stroke?

- Ask the person to stick out their tongue. If the tongue is crooked or goes to one side it is an indication that the person has suffered a stroke.

- The person won't be able to smile properly. Ask them to smile

- Inability to talk or speak coherently. Ask the person to repeat a complex phase.

- They will have difficulty raising both arms. Ask them to do this.

- The face goes white the lips may turn blue

Given that a person has suffered a stroke they have a maximum three hours to seek medical attention. If they can get to a hospital in this time the effect of the stroke can be reversed.

There are various reasons for strokes?

- Blockage of the arteries to the brain.
- Blood clots cutting of the flow of blood and oxygen to the brain.
- Rupture of the blood vessels in the brain.
- Very high blood pressure can also cause strokes.

Angina, a related illness is associated with panic and feeling like you are going to die. If affected you should immediately visit your doctor.

THE BLOOD PRESSURE STRESS CONNECTION

Stress alone can make a non-smoking, non-drinking person who is not on drugs, is not fat, is eating healthy food have a very high blood pressure. The good news is that stress can be overcome by exercise and at least one hour meditation daily.

BLOOD CIRCULATION

The circulatory system is made up of veins, arteries and tiny blood vessels delivering about 5.6 litres of blood rushing through our body.

White blood cells destroy invading bacteria. Red cells transport oxygen from the lungs to every cell of the body.

Platelets are denser cells whose job is to form clots to plug and repair damage to the blood vessel walls.

If the blood is deficient in iron then its proper function is not possible. Foods which contain iron are: lamb liver, salmon, tuna, poultry and oysters. For Vegetarians: Lentils, oats, cooked spinach, cooked chick peas, almonds, raisins, apricots, cooked beans.

There are many types of blood disease the most serious is leukaemia.

When damage is done to the bone marrow it will results in the production of abnormal cells which attack red blood cells. This condition is poorly understood.

The health of blood vessels is subject a proper diet.

If we consume refined foods and saturated fats a number of diseases will occur.

Heart attacks, strokes, arthritis, hardening of the arteries, blood clots which will prevent enough blood reaching the vital organs including the brain. All these potential dangers bring us back to the importance of the right diet and exercise.

One of the most dreaded conditions is stroke caused by brain aneurysm, a burst blood vessel inside the brain or a blood clot, which will cut off the blood supply to the brain. Brain cells will perish quickly if they are cut off from blood, which not only carries oxygen but also other nutrients which the brain needs.

If a stroke occurs on the left side of the brain then the right side will be affected and vice versa.

People can get stroke and heart attacks as a result of unbearable tension. Smoking and heavy consumption of alcohol can do the same.

People who are grossly overweight or in a bad physical condition can be affected by angina, a very painful condition caused by insufficient oxygen and blood reaching the heart, It might come suddenly when a great deal of physical activity is placed on the heart.

It can also happen when one is running fast up on a hill or after a heavy meal. If one is affected by this condition then it is essential to quickly call an ambulance with a paramedic who will treat you on the spot.

Doctors will probably then prescribe beta blockers.

A good diet and a lot of meditation will prevent this dreaded condition from arising.

SECTION 12. ALZHEIMER'S DISEASE

Alzheimer's is a modern disease, almost unknown before the 1930's, it affects the brain, which gradually deteriorates over the course of years. There is no medically accepted cure for Alzheimer's disease

Alzheimer's disease causes loss of memory, irritability, mood swings, difficulty speaking and a general inability for the sufferer to look after themselves.

In the final stages the patient finds it difficult to recognize even his close family. Death follows soon after.

According medical research, one of the main reasons for Alzheimer's is the presence of aluminium content in the food chain. Aluminium finds its way to the brain and causes plaques to develop. This blocks the way for communication between brain cells, decreases blood flow and the uptake of oxygen for vital brain function. Alzheimer disease can spread from cell to cell by means of a rough protein named TAU. The brain cells damaged by this protein reduce the brain's ability to retain memory and to reason.

Currently standard medical science does not offer a cure for Alzheimer's disease.

In order to postpone or avoid Alzheimer's disease we must avoid the following:

- Don't use aluminium or Teflon pots or pans, use only stainless steel pots.
- Don't drink any sort of liquid in aluminium containers.
- Avoid using aluminium foils for wrapping food.
- Avoid eating sugar, especially refined sugar as this will open

up the blood brain barrier and allow aluminium present in the blood to enter the brain. Sugar is a poison and which destroys brain cells.

- Avoid buying medicine or food products with the word 'ALUM' mentioned anywhere on the label.
- Don't buy antacid tablets containing aluminium, prolonged intake of aluminium not only increases the possibility of getting Alzheimer's but can cause serious liver or bladder damage as well.
- Use as little baking powder as possible.
- Reduce your blood cholesterol level to maximum of 5.5 as a high cholesterol levels in the brain clog the blood vessels and will contribute to the possibility of Alzheimer's. Cholesterol can clog not only the arteries, but the fine blood vessels of the brain as well and contribute to the onset of Alzheimer's.
- After lunch eat two pieces of Brazil nuts but no more than this.
  - Eat only whole meal, or black bread.
  - Use your brain as much as possible by reading, cross word puzzles and other mental exercises. Recently scientists came to the conclusion that people who use their brains more have less incidence of Alzheimer's disease.
  - Cut out smoking, alcohol and the consumption of refined foods.

Useful foods to reduce the aluminium content in the body are:

Liver, bran, beans, eggs, onions, nuts, sardines, tuna, salmon, assorted vegetables, apricots, asparagus, carrots, prunes, dates, potatoes, onion, garlic, cabbage, yoghurt and lemon juice.

Add to your diet three times week these supplements: One tablet of vitamins E, C, Niacin, B complex, Ginseng, Zinc and Ginkgo per day.

Lemon the best source of vitamin C. Mix it with a bit of apple juice and have after dinner.

Also, add to your diet one iron tablet three times a week.

Every day take some flaxseed or Udos oil as well as fish oil. Fish oil is the best food you can take for healthy brain function. Sardines are a good source of fish oil.

A shortage of some minerals in nature can also contribute to impaired brain function and general bad health. To supplement the lack of certain minerals in the soil and food take a teaspoonful of Colloidal minerals after breakfast. Colloidal minerals are available in liquid form from most health food stores.

A British study found that folate is one of the very best supplements for combating and preventing Alzheimer's. Folate can be taken in tablet form.

I would like to point out, if someone is already suffering from Alzheimer's then in addition to the above mentioned information, it is essential to exercise at least one hour a day. Exercises such as walking, swimming or indoor bicycle riding are beneficial. These will prevent or in the worst case slow down brain deterioration.

Linseed oil, which is actually flaxseed oil, is an excellent brain food. Linseed oil was first used and cultivated in the ancient Greek and Roman Empires and was considered a useful health product until the first world war. Take one table spoonful of linseed or flaxseed oil daily with food. Flaxseed or Udo's oil are rich in Omega 3 unsaturated fats. Fish oil and virgin olive oil are also highly recommended. Flaxseed oil can be applied to any food, for example on top of yourbreakfast cereal. Also, assorted nuts will keep the brain in good shape. In general the essential oils for brain function are; Omega 3 and Flaxseed oil.

By practicing these instructions you will give your brain a chance to be resist this horrible disease even if you have inherited this condition.

SECTION 13. DEPRESSION, STRESS AND PANIC ATTACKS

For most people life is full of difficulties.

When one cannot find a satisfactory solution to problems this triggers a depressive state in which people feel a sense of hopelessness, despondency and sadness. Divorce, loss of job, relationship issues, sexual issues, unable to pay the mortgage, anger, death or illness in the family, all can cause depression.

Depression is wide spread in the modern world. According the United nation health organization about thirty per cent of the population in the developed world has at one time or another suffered from depression. In the third world the rate is even higher.

In the mega cities of the USA New York, Chicago and Los Angeles more than fifty per cent of the population is occasionally affected by mental distress.

Depression can cause deep sadness, insomnia, loss of appetite, apathy, difficulty concentrating, tension, feelings of being inferior physically or mentally, feelings of anger, memory lapses, nausea, dry mouth, thoughts of death or suicide, nightmares, constant tiredness or difficulty sleeping or an excessive need for sleep.

People suffering from depression are likely to have high blood pressure, heart attacks, stroke, cancer, migraines and loss of sexual desire.

During depression the blood sugar level often rises which in the long run may lead to diabetes.

Depression in children and teenagers can cause youth suicide.

Depressed people often find relief in drinking, smoking and drug taking which ultimately damages their health.

Depression can deplete vital chemicals such as melatonin and serotonin which keeps the brain functioning properly.

Depression and stress can cause panic attacks, a very unpleasant physical and mental condition.

Panic attacks are extreme mental physical responses to a desperate situation. During panic attacks victims feel as if they are dying or going crazy, they may shake uncontrollably, have difficulty breathing or feel a strong desire to run or escape.

Once a panic attack starts it can last for hours at a time and they can reoccur months even years later.

One can safely say, that by having a panic attack the brain is doing itself a disservice, as it achieves the opposite to what it needs. In this state a person is not rational and is incapable of doing any physical or mental work.

During a panic attack repressed problems and phobias break through from the subconscious and wreak havoc on the unfortunate person. They are now very short of serotonin which normally prevents irrational thoughts from dominating the conscious mind. A horrifying fear of death floods the mind far stronger than any real life threatening situation.

During panic attacks a person may hyperventilate, (very rapid shallow breathing), which makes the panic attack worse.

The discomfort experienced in a panic attack can be so severe that some people are driven to commit suicide.

Our physiology is little changed from what it was thousands of years ago. In the past our lives were often in danger when fighting wild animals. In response to danger the brain produces adrenalin, cortisone and cortisol which gave us energy to fight or run. Adrenalin increases our metabolic rate and causes us to breathe fast. In a way the same thing happens in a panic attack. However the unfortunate person can't run away, nor can he fight the imaginary terror of death.

WHAT TO DO IN A PANIC ATTACK

In order to reduce the horrible feeling in intensity and duration place a paper bag over the mouth and nose and breathe in it slowly, then try to think of pleasant peaceful things. Do that for a few minutes. Then go for a long walk lasting at least an hour. While walking contract all muscles in the chest and arms to the count of five, then release them slowly.

To follow up take a medium breath not a deep one for the count five then hold your breath for the count of five, then exhale slowly.

Next, contract your muscles again to the count of five, and then release them slowly. Then repeat the above mentioned breathing exercises and keep on walking and breathing, but not too deep, then start all over again .This exercise should reduce the duration of panic attack considerably.

When reasonably calm try to meditate. If you are afraid to close your eyes then just shut them half way and breathe in and out softly.

A fear of death often arises in a panic attack. Feelings of inferiority, being unsuccessful and inability to face life overcome the mind. The mind loses control of aggression instincts and phobias from the subconscious take over. These feelings affect the brain in a negative way. In the case of losing someone close, one identifies with the loved one, to such an extent, that one feels that he or she is dying too. They may feel that they will be the next to die.

At one time or another all of us are afraid that we could lose someone we love, lose our job or health. Many of us look forward with fear to the future when we grow old, loose our beauty become sick and finally die.

Many people feel the world is cruel and uncaring: some of us feel overwhelmed by the struggle to survive and fall into depression and panic.

After suffering years of depression vital brain chemicals get depleted and we become oversensitive to such an extent, that even an unpleasant thought can trigger a panic attack.

One has to realize, that life is always associated with struggle, hardship, competition and natural disasters. That's life. Do what you can and accept what you can't change.

The answer is not to take things too seriously, when you have a panic attack, shake it off, fight back!

Do the various exercises described above. If you do all that, then each time you have a panic attack the duration will be shorter, finally it might only last a few seconds and in time it will disappear altogether, as your brain will adjust and look at life in a different way.

In order to avoid or reduce the possibility of depression and panic attacks, please follow some rules:

- Don't be fanatical about anything.
- Don't let worry get the better of you.
- Don't always demand success from yourself.
- Don't be fanatical about your looks and accept your age.
- Follow the golden middle way, treat yourselves with friendship and love, not aggressively and treat others the same way.
- Count your blessings.
- Exercise as much as possible, walking, swimming, etc. When you exercise, your brain will produce extra Serotonin.

- Take some multi vitamins twice a week plus one B complex twice a week and one B6 tablet every third day after breakfast, but not more than 100 mg.

The brain is very rich in fats. If it's get its fats from saturated sources such as lard, margarine oils manufactured with high temperatures then sooner or later it will become sick and degenerate causing various illnesses. One can reduce the effect of panic attacks depression and even the possibility of brain tumours, giving the brain the best fats available such as flaxseed oil, fish oil, virgin olive oils or assorted cold pressed oils.

In addition please take advantage of the previously mentioned healthy nutrition.

Meditate every day at least an hour.

Be patient with yourself, in time your brain will heal itself.

Reduce smoking, alcohol, stimulants such coffee, tea, coke drinks , chocolate, as even a small amount of those items can cause a new panic attack in sensitive people.

Have a warm shower at night before going to bed.

Do your deep breathing exercises at least three times a day

Don't work more than maximum of 60 hours a week.

Have a food allergy test; masked food allergies can cause mental problems and depression as can Candida.

Ask your GP for anti-depressant prescription.

Get rid of feelings of hatred and anger toward other people.

A whole banana will help you to increase your serotonin levels and make you feel better.

Niacin is helpful against depression as well against anxiety and confusion

STRESS

Life in the modern world creates a lot of stress. The same brain chemicals that were used thousands of years ago when we were in dangerous situations are present when we encounter stressful situations today. Lasting stressful situations increase blood pressure, blood sugar levels and reduces our body's ability to fight infections as well as cancer and can cause heart attacks.

The causes of Stress are many; here are a few of them

- Death of a spouse or a family member
- Overwork, (frequently occurs in Japan where some people work themselves to death)
- Financial worries, loss of a job
- Conflict within the family, or chronic sickness
- Aggressive neighbours
- Lack of rest
- Government bureaucracy
- Constant visits by friends, too much social life.

WHAT CAN WE DO TO REDUCE DEPRESSION AND STRESS?

Physical exercises, such as walking at least one hour a day, swimming, gardening, tennis are all helpful.

One hour before going to sleep have foods rich in serotonin such as a banana, cashew nuts, a couple spoons full of sesame seeds mixed with some fruit juice and tofu.

Don't have more than one cup of coffee and tea daily.

Count your blessings.

Wherever you can do some meditation, follow the information mentioned earlier; do at least 10 minutes of deep breathing daily.

Expose your body for about 15 minutes daily to the sun (unless your doctor advises you against it)

Avoid being overweight, give up smoking, drinking, drug taking.

Don't keep a grudge, be forgiving, help other people, don't be lonely and seek out friends and listen to music, if it is only possible sleep at least seven hours a day.

Banish feelings of anger and hatred against members of your family or friends, see their good points not only their negative ones.

If you feel stressed, nervous, before going to sleep tell yourself to relax and repeat under your breath that in the future you would like to be a more loving and more civilized person.

Start to sing under your breath and if you remember recite the words as well.

It helps you to go to sleep. If you wake up during the night, resume singing again until you fall asleep.

For the sake of peace and harmony reduce your criticism of you family members and friends.

To reduce depression drink only water, fruit juices, no soft drinks at all.

Omega 3 is very important, so have a tablespoonful of flaxseed oil mixed with some fruit juice every day.

Include in your diet walnuts, almonds, sesame seeds, banana, avocado, apple, some milk, fruit and vegetables daily, also some tofu, the juice of one lemon mixed with some apple juice. Have 5 eggs per week.

Three times a week eat some spinach, lentils, chick peas, beans, radishes, tomatoes and carrots.

THE DANGER IN GROWING UP

The most dangerous period in a person's life is childhood, when a naïve uncritical child, whose brain is not yet developed and can be told all sorts of stupid, unhealthy impractical illogical unscientific things by parents, teachers or guardians.

Unfortunately children will readily accept them. They then have a problem which can last a life time.

Growing up in broken homes is another danger, as well as brutal or abusive parents. Living in poverty, or neglect, bad company, a father or mother who constantly criticize the child making him feel worthless can have serious repercussions.

Even well off but uncaring parents can damage a child's mind.

The mental balance of the child eventually snaps giving rise to future depression, stress and in time mental disease.

Pestered by inner turmoil an unfortunate individual might transfer his or her aggression to other people which in some cases can result in excessive violence.

The saddest thing is that a child who suffers while living with violent parents or guardians will copy their behaviour when he grows up.

Although things have improved since ancient times we still live in a very hard and frightening world full of all sorts of violence including religious ones. So it is no wonder that almost half of the world's population is at times suffering from mental disorder.

It is not enough to have a large number of horrible diseases pestering us.

On top of it the human race is cursed with excessive aggression which we inherited from our ancestors the killer apes.

Every nation spends a sizeable income on armaments including the poorest nations. Terrorists kill in the name of God whose prime commandment was

> *"Thou shalt not kill"*

If we don't get destroyed by climate change or nuclear holocaust then perhaps in a hundred years or so no one will be allowed to have children unless they pass a test on how to raise them without harming their mental and physical health.

HAPPINESS

Happiness is hard to quantify however there are some interesting facts concerning a person's status and their longevity.

The death rate of divorced people is far higher than the married ones.

Widows and single people have far shorter lives than married people.

Happiness and health seem very much linked to one's social interaction.

SECTION 14. HEARING AND TINNITUS

The main symptom of Tinnitus is a constant ringing in the ear. Tinnitus is a problem affecting the central portion of the ear where thousands of tinny hair follicles are situated. Tinnitus has a number of causes: High blood pressure, diabetes, too much antibiotics and ear wax.

However the most frequent reason for Tinnitus is the damage to the inner ear caused by excessive exposure to noise over many years. It can also occur suddenly, when a person is subjected to one or many explosions. Soldiers returning from war often have ear damage.

On the whole we live in a very noisy world, and our hearing deteriorates much faster than that of our ancestors. This is especially true among young people who are exposed to a great deal of loud music. The noise level of a normal conversation is about 60 decibels. It has been proven that frequent exposure to noise above 80 decibels can cause loss of hearing. Music at rock concerts can reach 120 decibels and if someone is very close to the speakers he will suffer a permanent loss of hearing almost immediately.

Sound waves travel through the ear drum then through the set of tiny bones named the hammer and the anvil. The sound waves then enter the cochlea. In the cochlea there are thousands of tiny hair follicles which vibrate in response to sound. This movement sets off nerve impulses which are interpreted in the brain as sound. If we are subjected to constant excessive noise in time the hair follicles will break or be flattened.

People exposed to frequent noise over 100 decibels can also develop high blood pressure, ulcers and insomnia. It can even damage the heart.

It is especially damaging to pregnant women, in fact they will transfer the damage to their babies.

The government should appoint inspectors to visit pubs, dance halls and check noise levels. They will find that almost all places the noise level is far greater than it should be.

Unfortunately 98 per cent of people are not even aware of this health hazard. Within twenty years countless millions of people will not only suffer from tinnitus but other health issues because of this fashion of extremely loud music.

As was pointed out before, prolonged exposure to excessive noise causes damage to the ear, to be precise, to the tiny hair follicles in the cochlea. As a result a constant ringing noise arises.

The constant ringing in the ear can be so distressing that it has even driven some people to suicide.

Prolonged exposure to high noise levels also causes gradual loss of hearing. As yet modern medicine has no cure for tinnitus and hearing loss. However if one practices a number of exercises, which we call brain exercises, a partial cure is possible.

I would like to point out, that there are five different exercises and all of them have to be practiced for at least 20 minutes daily to be effective. The exercises are rather difficult, but instead of your condition getting worse every month, it will get better.

10 minutes here, 10 minutes there, whenever you find time. For the first month, 100 minutes per day. For the second month, 75 minutes a day will be OK. The following month, 50 minutes a day should do.

After this time you should keep on practicing at least 20 minutes a day, until all ringing in the ears stops.

The exercises are easy exercise, however one has the choice to do the exercises or let the tinnitus get worse. It should be a clear choice between tinnitus and hearing loss and getting better.

The following exercises will develop our powers of visualization and imagination which will be very helpful for other serious health problems as well.

We will learn to use the dormant electrical energy of our brain and be revitalized by the electric force surrounding our body. This electrical force is called the aura.

In our endeavour to heal ourselves we will also take advantage of the enormous cosmic energy field penetrating every part of our planet. In fact the cosmic energy field is all around us.

EXERCISE 1

In this exercise you will sit on a plain chair. Put your hands on your lap, then raise your physical hands and start massaging both your ears at the same time by pushing the palm of your hands tightly to your ears. Now push your hands up and down for about 20 seconds. Now take your hands away, as in this real exercise you will not use your physical hands. The healing work will be done only by using visualizations and imagination alone. Close your eyes and start massaging your ears with your both of your spiritual hands.

Just imagine that your hands are surrounded by a very dense concentration of bluish, or colored, energy field. This required energy will come from a number of sources, from your brain, from your aura and from incoming cosmic force.

Once you start the healing exercises your brain and immune system will help you from inside of your brain.

Start pushing your imaginary hands up and down, pushing the healing energy through your ears.

You have to visualize that the concentrated dense energy goes in through your ear and beyond that into your brain.

Visualize the energy massaging the damaged part of your inner ear. As we do this the blood circulation in and around the damaged inner ear increases removing the damaged and dying cells and replacing them with healthy ones. We do this exercise for about 10 minutes, on each side then stop. We open our eyes and get ready for the next exercise.

EXERCISE 2

In this exercise again we raise both of our physical hands and place both palms side by side so they cover a larger region. Move both hands over a single ear. Concentrate on one ear at the time with both hands raised. Let's say you start on the left side and start to massage your ear up and down, say for 20 seconds. Now remove your physical hands and let your mind take over and keep on moving both your imaginary hands up and down. Always close your eyes when you do any of the exercises.

Move your imaginary hands up when you inhale and down when you exhale, pushing the healing energy right into your ear. Keep doing this exercise for 10 minutes. Now do the same exercise on the right ear for 10 minutes. You are now ready for the next exercise.

EXERCISE 3

No physical contact will be needed in any of the exercises.

The healing activity will be done by the power of the mind. Close your eyes and start sending a heavy concentration of dense brain energy waves from the left side of the brain to the right side.

Visualize the energy as a horizontal column of energy pushing its way into your left ear, through the brain and out through the right ear. Think of the column as a wide laser beam traveling through the lower part of your brain under your skull. Do this exercise for 10 minutes, then reverse the order, in other words you will do the same again, except start on the right side and direct the energy flow to the left side. As you do this exercise, follow your brain waves with your inner eye from left to right and the reverse.

EXERCISE 4

Close your eyes and focus your attention to the inner center of your left ear, which in fact is very close to your brain. Now visualize the tiny blood vessels of the ear being saturated with hundreds of millions of tiny healing cells, nourishing cells and cells with special nutrients, all rushing forward to the inner ear where the damaged hair follicles are flattened and waiting for revival. Now in your imagination direct the increased flow of blood carrying all those nutrients mentioned before toward the tiny hair follicles, pushing its contents right inside the hair bulbs. By this action the tinny hair follicles will be revitalized and reinforced by the constant supply of new nutrients. The blood supply to the center of the ear will come through dozens of channels.

As you keep pushing the new supply of nutrients into the base of the tiny hair follicles they will become erect again and the noise in your ear will stop and your hearing will not deteriorate any more. This exercise should be practiced for 10 minutes on each ear.

EXERCISE 5

In this exercise you do not use your imaginary hands any more to massage your inner ear. This exercise is different from the others. The main component of this exercise will consist of using our brain power as well as the power of cosmic energy, which is in abundance all around us. Our brain is constantly producing electric energy which is vital to our heart and other body organs. In one part of the brain there is an electromagnetic section, which if stimulated, can attract cosmic energy forces. The cosmic energy will be absorbed by our brain and body and with that we will recharge ourselves. In order to do this exercise, we have to use various suggestions, close your eyes and visualize an energy field coming towards you. Imagine the energy field is a blue, green or purple cloud or wave slowly coming toward you. Let's say the wave strikes your left side and moves toward the center of your brain. The energy will go through the brain and exit on the other side, any part which is not absorbed will slowly dissipate. Now wait for about 10 seconds and reverse the process letting the energy enter from the right side, let it enter the ear and massage the inner ear, increasing the blood flow and healing the damaged hair follicles. It may be easier to visualize the energy flow as a child's cradle being rocked from left to right. Do this exercise for about 10 minutes.

As you push this energy through your ear follow the movement of the action with your inner eye. This exercise can be used to heal any part of your body, all you have to do is to direct the incoming energy to any part of the body where you feel discomfort or pain.

If you feel that you get enough energy flow from one side only that will be sufficient.

EXERCISE 6

Move your jaw up and down, like you would be chewing something hard. Do this 20 times, not more, once a day. Always close your eyes when doing the exercises.

If you wish you could spend less time on the above mentioned exercises, but then healing will take longer.

EXERCISE 7

From the upper left side of your brain send a column of energy to the right side of your brain and entering your ear canal sending healing energy to the center of your ear canal where the hair follicles are situated. This column of energy will massage your inner ear and promote healing. Do these for 10 minutes then reverse the procedure.

If you wish ask your doctors opinion or follow the same regime I did for which I received a one hundred per cent result.

Once you have healed your tinnitus avoid loud rock concerts or other noisy environments to prevent the condition from reoccurring.

IMPROVING HEARING

For hearing problems, chew flavoured chewing gum. Chewing exercises and stimulates the muscles close to the ear. Also, try a teaspoon of cinnamon mixed well with a half a cup of apple juice.

SECTION 15. EXERCISE

These days many people are too tired, too busy or simply not interested in doing exercise. However, in order to achieve a firmer, stronger, healthier body with the least possible discomfort there is nothing like some good old fashioned exercise.

EXERCISES FOR GENERAL WELL-BEING AND STATE OF MIND

Exercise or walk at least thirty minutes daily. Exercise increases blood flow and clean out the arteries. Exercise also releases endorphins and serotonin in the brain and helps depression.

FACE AND SKIN EXERCISES

Move your jaw up and down slowly stretching your facial muscles as you do. Do this exercise for about two minutes. Expand your face as if it was a balloon being blown up. Then let your face relax. Repeat about 20 times.

Both exercises will strengthen your facial muscles and add extra facial tissues, keeping your face not only younger looking, but also healthier. These exercises can be performed while you travel on a bus or a train. They can be also practiced in a dark cinema or at home.

MID BODY EXERCISES

Contract the muscles in your neck, then let them go and relax, then start all over again. Repeat about 50 times.

Contract the muscles in the upper part of your back. This will involve the front part of your chest muscles. Keep repeating the same movement about 50 times.

Contract the muscles of your stomach, and let them go again. Repeat

50 times. You will notice that by doing this exercise your lower back and your rectal muscles will also be involved.

EXERCISE FOR ARTHRITIS

If you suffering from arthritis or generally run down the next exercise will help to improve your well-being.

Close your fists tightly and contract the muscles on both arms for the slow count of five, relax and let your muscles go for the count of 10. Repeat this exercise for about 10 minutes. This will help to reduce inflammation. It is also beneficial to practice this exercise while lying in bed. This exercise will make you yawn a lot and put you in a relaxed state of mind ready to go to sleep.

EYE EXERCISES

To keep your eyes healthy please follow these suggestions:

Don't force or strain your eyes, keep them relaxed.

Don't stare at a fixed object for too long, keep your eyes in motion as much as possible.

If your work involves concentration for a longer period of time, then make a habit of looking away every 20 minutes preferably to an object in the distance and blink ten times.

If your eyes are tired or itchy, don't rub them just cover your eyes with the palm of your hand for a while. Also, try putting some water on your palms before apply them.

Eye Exercises:
- Roll your eye balls, without moving your head, upwards toward the ceiling, then reverse and look downwards as much as you can, leave your focus downwards for a couple of

seconds, then start again. Perform the exercise gently without force. Repeat 50 times.

- Roll your eye balls to the far right, leave them there for a couple of seconds, then reverse and look to the left. Repeat 50 times.

You can do these eye exercises while sitting on a bus. The above exercises will in time improve your sight.

TOWARDS UTOPIA

The utopian dream of a world without war, disease or starvation is alive and well. The difference being that in the past it was just a dream and unobtainable whereas now it is within our grasp thanks to improved medicine, better education and higher standards of living.

Darwin in his famous book "On the Origin of species" coined the term "Natural Selection" meaning *survival of the fittest*. In the distant past humanity was indeed fit, and needed to be to find food and shelter. However due to our current sedentary city life styles and lack of exercise we are not so fit anymore. Survival in today's modern society is now not so much an issue of physical fitness but of knowledge, education and positive mental attitude.

Science has given us many innovations to make our lives easier but science alone is not enough to make us healthy and happy. Goodwill and discipline are also needed. Science has not overcome inequality, war, pollution, crime and in some cases has even caused them. The nations of the world have to form a united front to prevent humanity from destroying itself. Countries can no longer live in ignorance and isolation when their neighbours are suffering or prospering. The world is now too small for that.

While we are no longer on the brink of worldwide nuclear destruction as we were in the cold war there are new even more pressing concerns that threaten us all. For example, the issue of global warming is real, whether it is manmade or natural. It is not unreasonable to expect major cities to be flooded if the ice caps melt or that living conditions in tropical areas will become unbearable forcing untold millions of people to migrate to cooler parts of the Earth where they may be not welcome.

Industrial pollution has already turned our planet into a greenhouse. Heat is trapped beneath clouds of smog causing the planet to heat up. Unless we want to drown in own waste products, the time has come to reduce pollution. The great oxygen producing forests of the world are disappearing at an alarming rate. In Brazil large tracts of the amazon jungle are burned off every day to make way for cultivation. The native Indians who have lived in these jungles undisturbed for centuries are forced off their land. The irony of the situation is that the whole exercise is futile as the soil is poor and can only support crops for a maximum of 3 years.

The time has come for the United Nations to stop Brazil and other countries from burning their forests and pouring millions of tons of pollution into the air. The United Nations should embark on a fast and desperate attempt to plant billions of trees all over the world, so that in time the new forests can at least partially absorb the excessive carbon dioxide and stop the world from warming up.

In third world countries like Sudan in Africa millions of children die of starvation while in first world countries like Australia, Canada, Western Europe and the USA there are enormous food surpluses. How can this inequality exist in a world where communication and transport has never been easier? The reasons are political and cultural and routed in history.

The current population of the world stands at seven billion. In 1960 there were 3 billion people on the planet. So the world population has more than doubled in 50 years. Should this rate of population growth continue the world will be under an incredible strain to feed itself. If Humanity wants to survive it is essential to introduce worldwide birth control and limit the number of children to 2 per family.

I hope the time will come, when every child that comes into this world will be planned and will be brought up by parents who have been tutored at schools in the art of being a parent and that we will have the resources to care for them.

Consumerism and built in obsolescence while driving profits up do so at a cost to the environment. We have become a throwaway society where nothing lasts longer than few years. Old products are discarded and become landfill. In short we are drowning in our own waste.

We have to sharply reduce our use of coal, petrol and other polluting materials. We can compensate by promoting the development of Hydrogen power, wind power, solar power, and both here on Earth and in space where enormous solar panels could be erected. The world should concentrate on renewable energy sources such as wind, tide, and geothermal power.

Tidal energy could be harnessed by building huge turbines in a number of locations on the continental shelves where the movements of the tides could be used to produce power.

Thermal power is a most promising option. An almost unlimited amount of heat could be extracted from the deep in the earth. Combined with water it can drive all the turbines of and generate electricity.

Public transport should be upgraded so that most people could leave their car at home most of the time they commute to work.

The hospitals of the first world are full of patients who need not be there had they lived a healthier life. These numbers can be reduced if governments were to ban the advertising of all harmful food products such as refined foods, alcohol and tobacco.

A strong United Nations police force would make it impossible to have dictators robbing their own nations of billions of dollars. They should be able to eliminate drug barons who are producing and pushing drugs around the world. This army could also make it impossible for regional wars or terrorists to exist anywhere in the world.

So there is no alternative, but a total control of all affairs by a world body, if Humanity is to survive.

ADDITIONAL INFORMATION

Hippocrates said:

"Let food be thy medicine and medicine be thy food."

Indeed this is the approach we use here. Through natural means I hope to provide a list of foods, supplements and regimes which will not only prevent but in many cases cure serious disease. If this sounds simple it is. You may find there is a degree of repetition in the list of item used to prevent or fight each disease. This is a good thing because the same foods can be used to prevent a variety of illnesses.

CANCER

Cancer can be reversed permanently through natural therapy without the need for chemotherapy. Chemotherapy not only kill cancer cells but healthy cells as well. After chemotherapy there is no guarantee that a recurrence of cancer will not occur at some stage in the future. Recurrence is unlikely if cancer treated through natural means. Chemotherapy introduces a toxic overload in the body which weakens our natural defenses to disease. Even if one decides to undergo chemotherapy it is advisable to combine it with natural therapies.

So what is natural cancer therapy? Natural cancer therapy is a series of diet and lifestyle choices designed to optimize health. I outline the components of natural therapy below.

The first step is to destroy the environment in which cancer can develop. This means eliminating all sugar and dairy products. Cancer cells cannot grow if we cut out those two items. By changing your diet you deprive cancer cells from the chance to develop. Replace the sugar and dairy products with fruits and vegetables.

Next stop eating processed and red meat. Examples of processed meat are ham, bacon, salami, sausages, etc. These meats are a major cause of bowel cancer, cholesterol buildup and high blood pressure. Replace the processed and read meat with lean meat e.g. chicken.

Next eliminate fried food from your diet, this includes deep fried fish and chips, fried chicken.

Next cut down of pasta, bread and white rice as these contain hidden sugar. Replace bread and pasta with other carbohydrate rich sources such as whole grains, legumes and fruit.

In general stay away from refined foods altogether. This means no eating food which comes in a tin, replace margarine with butter, etc.

Supplements

One should have two table spoon of flaxseed or Udos oil three times daily with a half a glass of carrot juice. Include three table spoons of vitamin C powder with the carrot juice. Other strong cancer fighting supplements are Ginkgo, inner health powder, magnesium, turmeric and grape seeds. All of which are available in your local health food store.

Anti-Cancer Foods

On one occasion I was invited to a party where I meet Patrick. At He was about 50 years of age. During our conversation he told me was a long term cancer sufferer. The last time he saw a doctor he was told that there was nothing further that could be done for him and that he had about three month to live. Shortly after that he came across a report by Professor Linus Pauling where he claimed that cancer can be cured through high doses of vitamin C powder. One table spoon morning, midday and night with meals mixed with carrot juice will do it. Patrick had nothing to loose so he followed the reports advice and after two months he was free of cancer. (Please read information about cancer diet on page number 85 and 86.)

Lemons are the most wonderful products of nature. The effect on the body is much stronger than any chemotherapy. The list of benefits is long: Lemons are effective against a wide range of bacterial and fungal infections, kill harmful parasites in the body, lower high blood pressure, fight depression, help nerve related disorders, effective against arthritis, kills cancer cells, reduces cholesterol, eliminate toxic metals from the body and reduce hypertension. Add the juice of one lemon to each meal.

Garlic is another strong natural cancer fighting agent. Have one piece of garlic with each meal.

Have three brazil nuts daily and three pieces of garlic with meals. Brazil nuts are a natural source of selenium which is missing from most western diets.

Parasitic causes of Cancer: Usually parasites live in the gut and intestines without causing any trouble. However the presence of isopropyl alcohol in the body triggers an explosion in the number of parasites in the body. These parasites attack the body and can cause cancer. The actual mechanism by which parasites attack the body occurs when the parasites die and produce ammonia. Ammonia is harmful to the body and brain and will interfere with sleep.

For more explanation on the effect of parasites in the body read Dr. Hulda Clark's book, *"The Cure for all Cancers"*

Garlic and onion will kill parasites as will cloves. Cloves can be purchased from your local supermarket. To eat cloves first grind them finely before mixing with yogurt.

Dairy products contain salmonella parasites, so in order to eat yogurt safely, mix in a tea spoonful of vitamin C powder before eating.

Garlic destroys cancer cells, reduces high blood pressure, kills harmful bacteria and parasites, prevents blood cells from sticking together and so reduce the possibly of strokes, heart attack and inflammation of the lungs.

If you taking garlic don't mix it with yogurt. Wait for three hours before eating yogurt.

Do not use cosmetic products as almost all of them are unhealthy especially the ones containing isopropyl alcohol. Check the packet labels for every ingredient on cosmetic and food products before buying them.

To safeguard your children give your pets an anti-parasite treatment.

Selenium will repair cells and fight cancer. The richest natural source of selenium is Brazil nuts. Selenium is an excellent anti-oxidant; it keeps the liver healthy, kills cancer cells, neutralizes heavy metals such as lead and mercury, reduces inflammation and arthritis and prevents eye cataracts if used regularly while one is still middle aged. Have two pieces of Brazil nut daily.

HOW TO CURE CANCER

- Eliminate sugar and dairy products from your diet. Cancer cells cannot exist without sugar and dairy products.
- No coffee or tea for a few months.
- No cosmetic products of any kind.
- No toothpaste
- No alcohol, or smoking
- No canned foods.
- No salt or cortisone,
- No white bread only rye bread.
- No hot or cold food or drink. no margarine
- Don't heat food in plastic containers
- No meat or any kind.

- No fried foods of any kind including chips
- No peanuts
- Drink six glasses of purified water a day, drink a glass of lukewarm water in the morning to remove waste products.. Don't keep water in plastic containers
- Clean your air conditioner filter once every month
- Walk at least twenty minutes a day
- No commercial juice of any kind except freshly squeezed orange juice
- Sleep as much as possible
- Use old fashioned land line phones not mobile phones which give off microwaves
- Two table spoons of inner health powder daily.
- Watch a funny movie such as 'Knock on Wood' with Danny Kay.
- Let go of any bitterness or anger and practice forgiveness to assist your recovery.
- Meditate for at least an hour daily to assist your recovery. Visualise millions of your cells destroying cancer. (see information on page 39)
- Practice deep breathing.

The anti-cancer diet

Your diet should be made up of 80% fruits and vegetables nuts, seeds, and fresh vegetable juices to assist the growth of building healthy cells. Until you are free of cancer don't have coffee tea and chocolate, drink purified water to avoid heavy metal and toxins from tap water.

Apples, pears, three pieces of Brazil nuts daily, walnuts, beans, cherries, cabbage, brussel sprouts, carrots, tomatoes, ginseng, cinnamon, spinach, onion, cranberry, apples, blueberry, broccoli, garlic, flaxseed, avocado.

Twice a day have two table spoons of flaxseed oil or Udos oil mixed with a half cup of carrot juice, two table spoon of vitamin C powder twice daily with a half cup of carrot juice. After the evening meal the juice of one whole lemon mixed with some carrot juice, lemon juice, vitamin C powder and flaxseed oil.

You can also destroy cancer by ordering a electronic parasite zapper from:

Arthur Doerksen BOX 2094. Abbotsford. BC.V2T3.X8 CANADA

Lemon juice is a very effective cancer fighting agent, it will reduce blood pressure and stress. Lemon juice can prevent strokes as it is a strong anti-coagulant. It destroys bad bacteria and kills parasites. Every day have the juice of one lemon with half a glass of apple juice or half a glass of water with one tea spoonful of honey.

STROKE AND HEART DISEASE

People affected by heart problems should take advantage of the following nutritional information: Have a handful of walnuts daily, as well some almonds macadamia nuts, sardines, almonds, avocado, sunflower and pumpkin seeds, oatmeal, blueberry, avocado, spinach, lentils, green tea, orange and lemon juice. On a slice of rye bread put two spoonful of olive oil.

Blocked blood supply to the brain will cause stroke which can kill or cripple a person. In some cases blindness is a side effect. In order to prevent this horrible situation it is essential to follow a number of preventive measures.

- Avoid fatty foods.
- Have multivitamins daily
- Walk or exercise one hour daily
- Have at least 7 glasses of water daily that can include a mild tea.
- Have 2 teaspoon of vitamin C powder daily mixed with half of glass of orange juice.

- Eat fish or sardine twice a week,
- Half an hour after dinner have 1 magnesium and 1 gingko tablet
- No smoking or drinking.
- More than 1 cup of tea and coffee daily
- Ask your doctor to check your blood pressure. (You may need blood thinners)
- Sleep at least 7 hours at night.
- Have a blood test once a year.
- 1 hour before bedtime, have a banana.
- Eat a lot of fruits and vegetables
- Have 2 table spoon of Udos oil with your morning meal.
- Drink only fresh fruit juice that you make yourself. (all other commercial juices contain large amounts of sugar, refined sugar is a poison)
- Have a piece of garlic in either the morning or night with your meal.
- Meditate at least a half an hour daily.
- Never eat fried foods, never eat food or drink liquids that are too hot or too cold. Have 3 pieces of Brazil nut daily .
- Don't eat red meat or white bread.
- Have 1 egg daily and 1 piece of garlic with dinner .
- If by misfortunate you are having a stroke then ask your doctor to immediately secure a wonder drug called Azlocillin

To lower cholesterol and fight cancer and arthritis have one tea spoon of cinnamon mixed with a little apple juice it is also anti-bacterial and anti-viral.

The healthy heart diet

In the morning have a bowl of 1 table spoon oat bran, 2 prunes, 2 dates, 2 brazil nuts, half an apple, and spoonful's of yoghurt.

For lunch: sardine with rye bread , or one egg with some avocado and rye bread.

For dinner: some chicken, salad , tomatoes, spinach, lentils , potatoes, a glass of orange juice.

One hour after dinner have a handful of ground walnuts, one banana and half a cup of blueberry.

- One hour before bedtime have one magnesium tablet with some water
- To avoid stroke have mainly a vegetarian diet.
- Have at least 7 glasses of water a day.
- Take two tea spoons full of vitamin C powder mixed with a half glass of apple juice daily.
- Have 1 vitamin B3 niacin tablet with your lunch daily. Niacin improves blood circulation in the brain.
- Have a piece of raw garlic with your breakfast. Garlic is a great anti-oxidant and will help to prevent blood clots.

HIGH BLOOD PRESSURE

Histidine will bring down blood pressure it is essential for the formation of myelin sheet which defends and the spinal cord it will protect against Alzheimer and Parkinson disease.

The low blood pressure diet

Fruits

Banana, melon, blueberry, pineapple, prunes, peaches, strawberry, nectarines, cherries, oranges. Oranges will reduce blood pressure, lower cholesterol

Nuts and Seeds

Raisins, dates, dark chocolate, flaxseed, sesame seed, sunflower seeds, pumpkin seeds, almonds, walnuts, pistachios, beets, garlic, turmeric, ginger. All nuts reduce high blood pressure. Raisins will lower your blood pressure it will reduce tension goods for the eye, the libido and dental health.

Meats, Fish and eggs

Chicken, turkey, eggs, sardines

Vegetables

Asparagus, red peppers, avocado, carrots, potato, salmon, beans, spinach, beetroot, broccoli

Other

Yoghurt, fish, oat bran, fish, mozzarella, orange juice, dark chocolate

Supplements to reduce high blood pressure

One ornithine tablet, tryptophan, magnesium, hawthorn tablets, coenzyme Q10

Have a warm shower before sleeping

STRESS, ANXIETY, DEPRESSION AND MENTAL ILLNESS

Foods with high salicylate content are a common cause of stress.

If you are affected by depression or other mental problems reduce your intake of the following food products: apricots, beans, broccoli, carrots, limes, dark zucchini, mangoes, passion fruit, radishes, prunes, raspberries, strawberries, cucumbers, mushrooms, olives, pepper, paprika, cinnamon, tomatoes, chestnuts, curry powder and coffee. Also avoid tobacco, drugs, alcohol, any food which contain artificial coloring and any sort of tea and white sugar. A little raw sugar is Ok, almonds and walnuts are fine.

Depression can be reduced by maintaining a balanced diet including nuts, sardines, salmon, herring, walnuts, eggs and brazil nuts, flaxseed oil, ginseng, vitamin B3, B6 and B12, Udos oil.

People who suffer from panic attacks should remove mushrooms from their diet.

All animals including people are infected by heavy metals such as cadmium, led, mercury, cobalt, nickel. Heavy metals are harmful to the body and can cause mental problems, depression and insomnia. One histidine tablet taken three times a week for two weeks will remove heavy metals from the body.

Stress can also be reduced by purifying the water we drink. Purchase a charcoal water purifier to remove chlorine and heavy metals present in tap water.

Zinc and vitamin C power is also helpful in removing heavy metals. Vitamin C powder will neutralize pesticides, herbicides and remove heavy metals like mercury. Zinc is very helpful to neutralize aluminium which is partly responsible for dementia and Alzheimer's disease.

One table spoons of apple cider vinegar mixed with a half of a glass water will remove toxins from your body as well raw garlic, carrots, green tea, avocado, apples, lemon juice, cabbage, turmeric, vitamin E and a handful of almonds

Amalgam tooth fillings contain mercury, ask your dentist to remove them.

Water, dirt, dust and paint often contain traces of lead which can cause lead poisoning.

Food products from China are often contaminated with mercury, a deadly poison. Some cosmetics, fish, red meats are also possible sources of mercury.

Cortisol is known to cause stress, memory loss and mood disorders and stress. Here is some information on how to reduce its effect:

Eat the following food products: Assorted nuts, berries, garlic, dark chocolate with 70% coco, green tea, salmon, 2 spoonful's of olive oil on a piece of rye bread and some paprika, turmeric. Those foods will produce essential gut bacteria and reduce your cortisol levels.

Bananas are good against depression. They also helps vision, bones and prevent kidney cancer. Bananas are rich in serotonin essential for good sleeping. Have two bananas per day not more.

For better mental health include in your diet omega 3, flaxseed oil, sesame seeds and walnuts.

If your serotonin levels are low eat beans, chicken, bananas, eggs and turmeric.

Dopamine is another organic chemical which plays a vital role in proper neuron transmitter function. To promote dopamine levels have the rolling foods and supplements: almonds, banana, dairy products, pumpkin seeds , sesame seeds, oats, dates, lemon ,blueberries, walnuts, avocado, turmeric, almonds, apples, sesame, sardines, salmon, tomato, chicken, vitamin B12, C, E, zinc, Udos oil.

Monosodium glutamate is harmful to the brain. Most if not all Chinese foods contain monosodium glutamate to some degree.

DEMENTIA AND ALZHEIMER'S

Dementia, which eventually leads to Alzheimer, is a horrible deadly disease. However if we follows the information presented below it can be avoided.

I could write pages about that terrible condition but I prefer to summarize and give you the most reverent points:

- Never drink any sort of soft drinks; they contain aluminium, which is a poison to the brain. The only safe drink is water or cold pressed orange carrot or apple juice.
- No smoking or drinking, no more than one coffee or one tea a day.
- Only use stainless pots for cooking never aluminium ones. Aluminium is a major cause of Alzheimer's disease.
- Don't use aluminium foil to wrap food.
- Sharply reduce your intake of sugar. Sugar is a poison
- All nuts and seeds, sardines, tuna, salmon, apricots, carrots, prunes, onion, garlic, yoghurt with lemon juice, asparagus, orange juice, cherries, avocados, eggs, almonds, walnuts, sesame seeds, sunflower and pumpkin seeds are especially helpful.
- Ten minutes sunshine and thirty minutes exercise daily is a must.
- Two tablespoons of flaxseed or Udos oil it's an excellent source of Omega 3 which is essential for proper brain function.
- For vitamins; one multi vitamin daily, zinc and foliate tablet three time a week.
- To boost the brain performance, have a one Bioglan turmeric anti-inflammatory tablet daily.
- Twenty minutes daily meditation will be one of the strongest anti Alzheimer remedies
- Have a cup full of blueberry and two spoonful of coconut oil daily. For oil only use virgin olive oil.

If one is already suffering from Alzheimer it is essentials exercise at list one hour daily. Avoid buying goods which contain aluminium as this is dangerous for the brain. Also, stay away from antacid tablets containing aluminium. Avoid fatty food which clogs your arteries. You should not have a cholesterol level of more than 5.5.

Foliate deficiencies can cause Alzheimer's, strokes, spinal cord problems. Take folate tablets. Natural sources of foliate include: lentils, avocado, and chick peas.

Ginkgo biloba and blue berry are helpful against Alzheimer, stroke, anti-dementia. They increase blood flow to the brain, are good for the eyes yoghurt reduces anxiety

SLEEP DISORDERS

If you have difficulty sleeping, don't watch more than three hours of television a day and especially not two hours before bed time. Ornithine capsules can also be helpful in promoting normal sleep patterns. These can ordered online from health supplement web sites such as www.vitacost.com . Take two capsules the first night then one more each night up to 6 maximum per night.

To sleep better have the following foods:

Chicken, chamomile tea, almonds, walnuts, banana, rice, yoghurt, blueberry, spinach, oatmeal, eggs, turmeric and ginger, nuts and seeds, rice, potatoes, banana, cherry, chamomile tea, green tea, cranberry and pomegranate juice. Pomegranates have strong anti-cancer, anti-inflammation properties and are good for the prostate, it will lower blood pressure, reduce arthritis, heart disease, fungal infections.

Proper serotonin levels in the brain are important for sleep. Melatonin is a brain hormone which helps us sleep. Normally melatonin levels are high at night and low during the day. Melatonin levels drop if we are subjected to light, especially the blue light wavelengths which are emitted from televisions and computer screens. Melatonin tablets are available from chemists.

MALE HEALTH

Excessive consumption of dairy products can harm the male prostate. Excess dairy products will reduce the sperm count and libido. Dairy products also cause the production of mucus which is bad for people suffering from bronchitis and cancer.

Testosterone is hormone which is directly related to male libido and erectile dysfunction. To boost testosterone levels naturally eat the following: potatoes, macadamia nuts, raisins, brazil nuts, almonds, pine nuts, ginger, eggs, avocado, spinach, yogurt, blueberry, apricot, coconut, onion, garlic, banana, porridge, cherries, dates, lemon, watermelon, pineapple, flaxseed, ginger, ginseng

Supplements to boost testosterone levels include: vitamin C, vitamin D, vitamin B3 (niacin assist blood circulation), vitamin E and L Arginine. L arginine is an anti-toxin; it lowers blood pressure, helps erectile dysfunction, depression and is good for improving vision.

Erectile dysfunction is a common ailment in men and can be alleviated by taking the rolling foods and supplements: flaxseed, pomegranate, watermelon, ginger, dark chocolate, pine nuts, salmon, eggs, red peepers, tuna, avocado, spicy food, cherries, onion, garlic, lemon, blueberry, spinach, banana, porridge, beetroot. Vitamin B12, magnesium, panax ginseng and Gingko

DIABETES

Vitamin E is helpful in preventing and controlling diabetes. Stay away from food products which contain benzoic acid. Check the labels on the packet. Eat pumpkin, sesame seeds, almonds, sunflower seeds, cashews, spinach and one magnesium tablet per day.

BONES AND ARTHRITIS

- To improve bone density and to prevent breakages have three tablespoons full sesame seeds with breakfast. Sesame seeds are the richest source of calcium.
- Have 6 pieces of prunes daily .
- Go walking at least a half an hour daily. Dancing and playing golf are also beneficial.
- Against arthritis eat sardines, nuts, herring, garlic, oranges, lemon, blueberry oat bran, cherries, green tea, garlic, ginger and turmeric,
- supplements to treat arthritis: gingko biloba, krill oil, vitamin D, zinc, vitamin E, omega 3 and pine bark extract
- cut down on sugar

Every person over the age of 50 needs extra calcium and the best source is not milk, (of which you must drink far too much to get the calcium you need), but sesame seeds. Three table spoons mixed with your morning meal. Note that elderly people should not use calcium tablets as they do more harm than good. Older people cannot absorb the calcium in these tablets. Instead they should have three soup spoonful's of sesame seeds with half a glass of milk which will be readily absorbed by the body. Baked beans, hazel nuts, dried figs are also rich in calcium.

OBESITY AND WEIGHT ISSUES

- Don't eat margarine, or fried chips as they are full of saturated fats which can clog the arteries.
- Have some nuts various seeds, and sardines every second day.

HEARING LOSS

Foods for better hearing

Brazil nuts (3 pieces daily), fish, almonds, eggs, chicken, oranges, apricot, melon, yoghurt, sesame seeds, walnuts and lentils.

Reduce your intake of fatty foods, antibiotics, dairy products and cold food or drink.

There is evidence to suggest that vitamin B3 Niacin produces better hearing. Foods rich in Niacin are: fish , eggs, beets and sunflower seeds

Supplements for better hearing

Vitamin B3 (niacin) B12, vitamin D, vitamin E, magnesium and Udos oil.

If you have an ear infection, ask your GP for Sofradex.

SKIN

For skin health eat pineapple, dark chocolate, cranberries, apple cider vinegar, 2 brazil nuts, coconut oil.

If you have skin problems stop using cosmetic products like deodorants, mouthwash, perfumes. Do not use hair sprays. Most cosmetic products contain propyl alcohol

TEETH AND GUMS

After eating always rinse with water in order to avoid gum infection. Also massage your gums for 20 seconds as inflamed gums can damage your heart. Please note that sugar is a poison and will destroy your teeth.

INFLAMMATION

A handful of almonds daily will reduce inflammation. Almonds are also good for the heart, prevent clogging of the arteries and prevent Alzheimer's.

Foods to reduce inflammation: blueberries, cherries, apple, papaya, cabbage, corn, pineapple, coconut, cranberry, spinach, tomato, broccoli, capsicum, garlic, ginger, flaxseed, walnuts, ginger, turmeric, green tea and cranberry. Take one magnesium tablet daily, flaxseed oil and cortisol cream.

Magnesium is anti-inflammatory and reduces blood pressure.

THE DANGERS OF SUGAR

Excessive sugar causes a wide range of health issues. Without exception all commercial juices are full of sugar and sugar is a poison. The only healthy commercial drink is fresh pressed fruit juices such as apple, orange, carrot juice.

VISION

After the age of 65 our eyesight deteriorates. There is a danger of macular degeneration which if left untreated can lead to blindness. In order to avoid macular degeneration see an eye specialist and ask for MacuVision tablet. Having a handful of walnuts daily will also help to keep your eyes healthy, as well juice of a whole lemon mixed with some apple juice.

To improve eye sight take the following: the juice of one lemon mixed with apple juice, almonds, pistachios, pacific salmon, dark grapes, one hardboiled egg daily, orange juice, wheat germ, blueberries, unsalted butter, two pieces of brazil nuts daily, avocado, spinach.

Avocados will protect your eyes, reduce cholesterol, fight cancer, arthritis, good for the heart, it has 40 minerals and vitamins.

Do eye exercises to strengthen your eyes.

Supplements for better vision: Vitamin A, E, daily one tea spoonful of vitamin C powder, one table spoon of Udos oil, ginkgo biloba, one lutein tablet daily and krill oil.

All these items will help against macular degeneration, especially a handful of walnuts daily.

To reverse macular degeneration have the following over a period of three days: One tea spoon of vitamin C powder daily, pistachios, ginkgo biloba, flaxseeds, ginger, sage and garlic.

DIGESTION

Taking 6 pieces of prunes daily will prevent constipation, indigestion and prevent urinary tract infection. Prunes are rich in iron and vital in building muscle, preventing blood clots, strengthening bones, reducing inflammation, preventing cancer, reducing blood pressure and fighting depression.

Bacillus pylori is a bacteria usually ingested though polluted water which lives in the gut and causes illness. Bacillus pylori if left treated can cause stomach problems. The recommended allopathic treatment is antibiotics. Repeated doses of antibiotics will kill the pylori bacteria but will also kill good bacteria in the gut.

To kill the pylori bacteria naturally eat the following foods: Manuka honey, cranberry juice, green tea, garlic, turmeric, ginger, cinnamon, ginseng, sauerkraut, apricots, banana, yoghurt, asparagus, inner health powder and one spoonful of apple cider vinegar with a glass of water daily.

For stomach acid have oatmeal, ginger, banana, melon, chicken couscous and asparagus.

HEADACHE AND MIGRAINE

Fermented foods like vines, pickled herrings, very ripe cheeses, sausages, and antihistamine can cause migraine headaches in sensitive people.

To treat migraine have seven glass of water daily, one multi B vitamin and two magnesium tablets daily.

SINUS PROBLEMS

Carrots, eggs, pumpkin seeds, tomatoes, nuts, pistachios, almonds, two spoonfuls of apple cider vinegar with a half of cup water a little bit of honey, turmeric tablets, zinc, vitamin A and L arginine.

LIVER AND KIDNEY FUNCTION

Magnesium and vitamin B6 keep the kidneys healthy. To clean the liver take L Arginine, assorted nuts.

FLU AND COLD

One tea spoonful of cinnamon daily mixed with half a glass of water and a teaspoon of honey is helpful to fight influenza and flu. Every day we pick up viruses, parasites, and all sorts of germs with our hands and fingers. Wash your hands and face each time you go home to avoid catching a cold or flu. In order to avoid infections don't put your fingers in your mouth unless you wash your hands thoroughly.

GENERAL HEALTH

Never drink cold water or water with ice with your meals at it will compress your food and make it very difficult to digest. Don't have very cold or very hot food as they can cause cancer on the long run.

Never drink commercial bottled water as it is contaminated by bacteria and harmful chemicals.

Don't smoke

Don't drink alcohol

Don't eat white bread, it is full of sugar.

Don't eat processed meat and cut down on read meat. Cooked chicken is fine.

Never heat food in the microwave in a plastic container. When put in a microwave the heavy metals in the plastic will mix with the food. Use ceramic containers instead.

All commercial fruit drinks contain a high level of sugar so drink them in moderation. The healthiest drinks are fruit juices which you make yourself.

If you have skin problems stop using cosmetic products like deodorants, mouthwash, perfumes. Do not use hair sprays. Most cosmetic products contain propyl alcohol which will cause the uncontrolled proliferation of parasites within the body.

Avoid foods which have been artificially coloured, such as ice cream, biscuits.

Every day take two bananas, two pieces of Brazil nuts, two spoonful's of flaxseed oil with water. One banana an hour before bedtime will help you to sleep.

Here is some information on chemical substances which can negatively affect various parts of your body:

Brain:	Alcohol, smoking, sleeping tablets
Lungs:	Petrol fumes, kerosene fumes and smoking.
Eyes:	Methyl alcohol, Cortisone, Viagra.
Heart:	Anti-depressants.
Kidneys:	Aspirin.
Liver:	Paracetamol, smoking and alcohol.

Toxic Overload In our modern world there are thousands of chemicals present in our water supply. In order to neutralize their harmful effects we should include one Zinc, one vitamin B3, and two magnesium tablets three times a week in our diet.

For better **blood circulation** blueberry, dark chocolate, oranges, avocado, ginger, garlic, pumpkin seed.

To prevent **hair loss** have vitamin B3 niacin, B12, C, D, E and zinc all of which are available at your local chemist

Parasites Every person to some extend is infected by parasites live in the body. The body destroys most but not foreign parasites. When these parasites die the by product is ammonia which attacks the brain and it makes it difficult to sleep well. One third of a tea spoonful of **L Arginine** will neutralize ammonia. Note that it will also bring down blood pressure, restore lost libido.

If you find that your health problems do not respond to conventional treatment then try Hulda Clark's electronic zapper treatment. As well as killing parasites the zapper is useful against Headaches, Depression, Parkinson, Alzheimer, Psoriasis, Arthritis, Fatigue and Herpes.

Zinc will also remove cadmium and other dangerous metals. It will help people with diabetic and prostate problems, sexual development in boys. Pregnant women should include zinc their diet. Zinc tablets are available in pharmacies. Food sources of zinc: Beef, lamb, salmon, bran flake, sunflower seeds, cashew nuts, oat bran and nuts.

Turmeric treats multitude ills. It is rich in potassium, magnesium, vitamin B6 and E. It is helpful against all type of disease. Turmeric will reduce cholesterol, inflammation, arthritis, asthma, heart problems, prevent Alzheimer's, diabetic condition, psoriasis, memory loss, fight cancer, inflammation, Parkinson, depression, macular degeneration, pylori. Turmeric is good for the heart and eyes. Turmeric has been called the world's strongest natural chemotherapy and stops the methylation of cells which is the precursor to cancer

Lemon Juice is a strong cancer fighting agent. It will also reduce blood pressure and stress. Lemon juice can prevent strokes as it is a strong anticoagulant. It destroys harmful bacteria. Everyday have the juice of one lemon half a glass of apple juice or water with one teaspoon of honey.

Omega 3 and 6 is vital for good health. The following products contain omega 3 and 6:

UDOS oil, brazil nuts, pumpkin seeds, sesame seeds, avocado and walnuts.

Garlic is anti-viral, anti-bacterial, anti-fungal, prevents cancer and reduces heavy metal toxins.

Vitamin C prevents cancer, hypertension, stroke, remove heavy metal, lowers blood sugar, reduces inflammation, destroys the helical bacterium and lowers blood pressure.

L histidine is essential to keep the myelin sheet which covers all the blood vessels especially in the spine. it is anti-Alzheimer, anti-Parkinson, anti-inflammation, anti-arthritis, it is also bring down high blood pressure.

Sesame seeds have anti diabetes properties, reduces blood pressure, cholesterol, anti-inflammatory, anti-cancer, good for the liver, reduce arthritis, good for the bones, eyes, lungs, skin. Sesame seeds contain tryptophan to make serotonin, reduce depression.

Pumpkin seeds contain tryptophan which helps sleeping, eases depression, good for the bones, anti-fungal, diabetes, good for the kidneys. Pumpkin seeds contain vitamin E and zinc.

Beetroot juice is good in reducing inflammation, diabetic conditions, for the brain, eyes and arthritis

Magnesium prevents Alzheimer's, reduces high blood pressure, and prevents diabetes. Magnesium can be found naturally in pumpkin, sunflower seeds, spinach, almonds, sesame seeds, avocado, blueberry, garlic, beetroot, turmeric, green tea and sauerkraut.

Pine bark extract will reduce blood pressure, fight arthritis, improve blood circulation, promote proper brain function and hearing, reduces inflammation, fight cancer and heart disease.

Folic acid is essential to good health and can be found in foods such as lentils, chick peas and avocado.

Ginger lowers blood sugar, cholesterol, good for the brain, reduces muscle pain and arthritis.

BIBLIOGRAPHY

Budwig, J. The Fat Syndrome

Erasmus, Udo. Fats that Heal Fats that Kill

www.ingramconten .com/pod-product-compliance
Lightning Source L_C
Chambersburg PA
CBHW070238230526
45470CB00002B/449